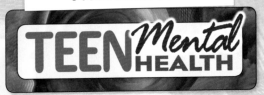

Teens and ADHD

Carla Mooney

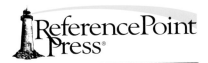

ReferencePoint
Press®

San Diego, CA

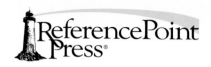

© 2017 ReferencePoint Press, Inc.
Printed in the United States

For more information, contact:
ReferencePoint Press, Inc.
PO Box 27779
San Diego, CA 92198
www.ReferencePointPress.com

LIBRARY OF CONGRESS CATALOGING-IN-PUBLICATION DATA

Names: Mooney, Carla, 1970- author.
Title: Teens and adhd / by Carla Mooney.
Description: San Diego, CA : ReferencePoint Press, Inc., 2017. | Series: Teen
   mental health series | Audience: Grade 9 to 12. | Includes bibliographical
   references and index.
Identifiers: LCCN 2016040558 (print) | LCCN 2016041410 (ebook) | ISBN
   9781682821206 (hardback) | ISBN 9781682821213 (eBook)
Subjects: LCSH: Attention-deficit disorder in adolescence--Juvenile
   literature. | Attention-deficit disorder in
   adolescence--Treatment--Juvenile literature.
Classification: LCC RJ506.H9 M656 2017 (print) | LCC RJ506.H9 (ebook) | DDC
   616.85/8900835--dc23
LC record available at https://lccn.loc.gov/2016040558

CONTENTS

Distracted and Unfocused

Throughout most of her teen years, Sarah Shearman struggled with undiagnosed attention-deficit/hyperactivity disorder (ADHD). As early as fourth grade, Shearman found it difficult to focus as she tried to complete her homework in her room. "I'd be in there for hours and I wouldn't get anything done," she says. "Sometimes I'd fill entire pages with doodling." Frustrated and anxious, she also felt an overwhelming urge to move around. At the time, Shearman complained in a diary entry, saying, "My mother wants me to settle down and do my homework! Doesn't she understand that I need a break? I need to get out of my room! But she won't let me!"[1]

In school, too, Shearman felt as if she needed to get up constantly and move. "I remember being in class and feeling like I was going to explode if I couldn't get out of my seat," she says. "My heart rate would go up. I felt like I was crawling out of my skin." To escape, Shearman would ask the teacher if she could leave the classroom. She explains, "I'd ask to go to the washroom, and then I'd just take off. I had my route. I'd go up and down the staircases and halls. I'd talk to other kids I met. Anything to get away from that feeling."[2]

For years, Shearman's ADHD went undiagnosed. She found it difficult to explain what she was feeling and experiencing because she did not understand that her mind functioned differently from those of other students in her class. Her parents, teachers, and doctors attributed her symptoms and difficulty focusing to anxiety. "They thought I couldn't focus because I was anxious.

Really, I was anxious because I couldn't focus. I tried to tell people that, but they didn't listen. That's why it took so long to get the right help,"[3] Shearman recalls. Eventually doctors diagnosed her with ADHD when she was a senior in high school.

ADHD is one of the most common neurodevelopmental disorders that affect children and teens, influencing the way their brains grow and develop. According to the Centers for Disease Control and Prevention (CDC), 10.2 percent of children ages five to seventeen are diagnosed with ADHD in the United States. For many of these children and teens, the symptoms caused by ADHD will continue into adulthood and may affect their performance at work and their relationships with family and friends. "Early in my career, I had trouble focusing, and I was always interrupting my teammates," says Major League Baseball player Shane Victorino. "My coach approached me and asked if I had trouble focusing when I was growing up. I told him I had ADHD as a kid, but thought that I had outgrown it. After that conversation, I went to the doctor, who confirmed that I still had ADHD."[4]

> "I remember being in class and feeling like I was going to explode if I couldn't get out of my seat."[2]
>
> —Sarah Shearman, diagnosed with ADHD as a child

Misunderstood and Misdiagnosed

Though ADHD presents differently in each person, common symptoms include impulsivity, inattentiveness, and hyperactive behavior. For many people, these symptoms are misunderstood and misdiagnosed. Parents and teachers often believe that a teen with ADHD needs to work harder or stop being lazy about completing schoolwork. They insist that a teen cannot have a problem with attention because he or she can focus intently on certain activities, such as watching television or playing video games. And because everyone feels distracted or unfocused at times, many people do not understand that ADHD is a real medical condition. "ADHD manifests itself in ways that everyone can relate to, so they conclude that there is nothing special about ADHD and that people with ADHD are just making excuses for themselves,"[5] says Douglas Cootey, author of an award-winning blog about ADHD.

ADHD is not, however, a simple problem of misbehaving or being lazy. Research has found that the brain of a person with ADHD works differently from that of a person without the disorder. This means that people with ADHD cannot, for example, will themselves to pay attention or stop feeling the urge to move.

When left undiagnosed and untreated, ADHD can have a significant impact on sufferers' lives. They may struggle in school and at work when their symptoms interfere with their ability to perform. ADHD can also cause stress and conflict at home when teens and parents clash. Teens with ADHD also face a higher risk than their peers of accidents, teen pregnancy, drug and alcohol abuse, and smoking.

Conquering ADHD

When ADHD is identified early and treated, a person with the disorder can lead a full and productive life. Many people with ADHD have gone on to be very successful. Well-known people—in addition to Victorino—who have been diagnosed with ADHD include actor Channing Tatum, singer Justin Timberlake, and Olympic swimmer Michael Phelps. After being diagnosed at age nine, Phelps underwent treatment, including medication and behavior therapy, to manage his ADHD. With treatment and the support of his family, Phelps was able to focus his energy on swimming. He became the most decorated Olympian of all time, achieving the amazing feat of winning 28 medals, 23 of which are gold, over his career.

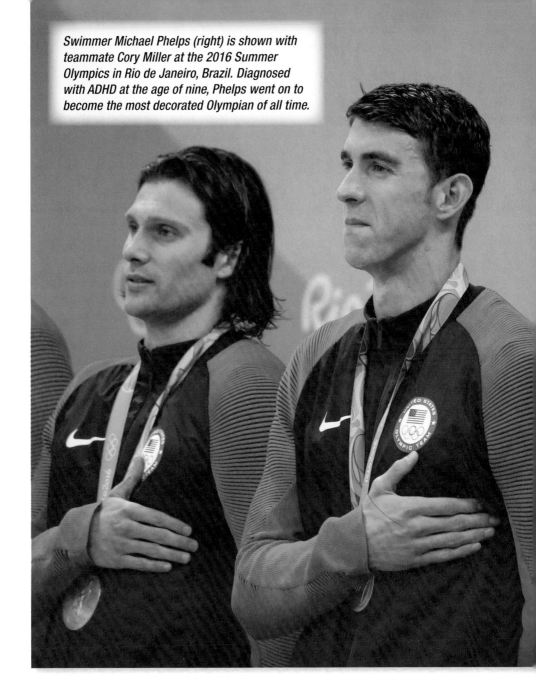

Swimmer Michael Phelps (right) is shown with teammate Cory Miller at the 2016 Summer Olympics in Rio de Janeiro, Brazil. Diagnosed with ADHD at the age of nine, Phelps went on to become the most decorated Olympian of all time.

Patricia Quinn, a developmental pediatrician and founder of the National Center for Girls and Women with ADHD, stresses the importance of an accurate diagnosis and effective treatment. "Most people with ADHD are smart; they are trying," she says. "If we diagnose and treat the disorder, these same individuals can be very successful."[6]

CHAPTER ONE

What Is ADHD?

Everyone has problems from time to time sitting still or pay-ing attention. People occasionally find their thoughts drift-ing at school or work or allow themselves to give in to impulsive behavior. For some people, however, problems with inattention, hyperactivity, and impulsiveness are serious enough to interfere regularly with daily life. These people may have ADHD.

A Chronic Brain Disorder

ADHD is a neurodevelopmental disorder that impacts a person's emotions, learning abilities, self-control, and memory. Like many other diseases and disorders, ADHD is a chronic (long-lasting) condition. For many people, ADHD symptoms emerge in child-hood and continue into adulthood. Although it cannot be cured, it can be alleviated with treatment.

ADHD affects every person differently, with some symptoms being more noticeable in some people than in others. Children with ADHD often appear hyperactive and impulsive, more so than children of the same age and developmental level. They have a hard time reining in their physical activity and appear overly active. They might also have difficulty controlling what they say, blurting out comments that are tactless or vocalized at the wrong time.

In addition, many children and teens with ADHD often struggle to pay attention. They may have trouble focusing on a task and shifting attention from one task to another. They may become easily distracted and appear extremely disorganized. "I felt differ-ent starting in 2nd grade because I just couldn't control my body movements and I was constantly talking," says twenty-five-year-old Andrea Goodell.

Even in school situations where I knew it was important to listen and pay attention, I found that I just couldn't help myself; I had to move, daydream or talk to other kids. It just made me upset and frustrated because I felt as if my body reacted in a different way than I wanted to. I would know the answer to a question, and I'd raise my hand and before I was called on I'd blurt out the answer even though I wanted to wait to be called on.[7]

Typically, ADHD symptoms begin in childhood, often emerging between the ages of three and six. With children this young, it is often difficult to tell the difference between typical preschooler behavior and symptoms of ADHD, but parents might notice that their toddler cannot stay still or that their preschooler is extremely impulsive. By the time a child enters elementary school, parents and teachers may be better able to spot the signs of ADHD. A child may be more impulsive and disruptive in class than same-age peers or less capable of sitting still and focusing on a lesson. "My 12-year-old stepson, Chase, was diagnosed with ADHD in kindergarten," says disability advocate Michelle Nielson from Twin Falls, Idaho. "He wasn't like most kids who'd sit in their seat and follow direction. He was always getting time-outs, always in trouble because he couldn't control himself. He was hitting other kids. When you're told your kindergartner is suspended, it's devastating. We'd just thought, he's a rambunctious little boy. We didn't know much about ADHD."[8]

> "I felt different starting in 2nd grade because I just couldn't control my body movements and I was constantly talking."[7]
>
> —Andrea Goodell, a young adult who has ADHD

People of varying intellectual abilities can all experience the symptoms of ADHD. Having ADHD does not make a person less intelligent than others. In addition, ADHD can affect people of all ages. Although most people are diagnosed with ADHD as children, others do not learn that they have the disorder until their late teens or in adulthood. And more than 75 percent of people

ADHD by Age and Gender

ADHD is the most common neurobehavioral disorder diagnosed in children and teens in the United States. According to the Centers for Disease Control and Prevention, 9.5 percent of young people aged four to seventeen have been diagnosed with ADHD. However, this varies by age and gender. The prevalence of ADHD was highest among youth between the ages of twelve and seventeen. And among all age groups, boys were much more often diagnosed with ADHD than girls.

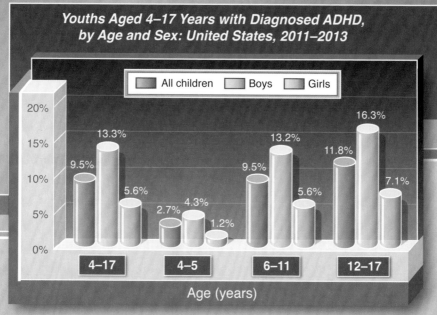

Youths Aged 4–17 Years with Diagnosed ADHD, by Age and Sex: United States, 2011–2013

Legend: All children | Boys | Girls

4–17: 9.5%, 13.3%, 5.6%
4–5: 2.7%, 4.3%, 1.2%
6–11: 9.5%, 13.2%, 5.6%
12–17: 11.8%, 16.3%, 7.1%

Age (years)

Source: Centers for Disease Control and Prevention, "Association Between Diagnosed ADHD and Selected Characteristics Among Children Aged 4–17 Years: United States, 2011–2013," May 2015. www.cdc.gov.

diagnosed with ADHD while in school continue to experience symptoms as adults. Their symptoms, however, may change as they grow older, with many people who were hyperactive and impulsive as children outgrowing these symptoms but still having problems with inattention and focusing.

Three Types of ADHD

There are three main types of ADHD: predominantly inattentive, predominantly hyperactive-impulsive, and combined. The type of ADHD a person has is diagnosed according to the symptoms primarily experienced. People with predominantly inattentive ADHD often find it very difficult to pay attention to details and sustain attention. They appear not to listen and have a hard time following conversations. They make careless mistakes and find it difficult to follow instructions. People with inattentive ADHD may be very disorganized and lose things frequently. They may become easily distracted and forgetful in daily life. Because they find it difficult to focus, people with inattentive ADHD may find themselves avoiding tasks that require sustained concentration and mental effort. Although people with the inattentive type of ADHD may also have some problems with hyperactivity or impulse control, their main symptoms revolve around inattention.

Dana Olney-Bell is a sixth grader with predominantly inattentive ADHD. Although she is smart and creative, she finds that she has to work harder than others in her class to pay attention and memorize information for tests. "In math, science, and art, I'm quicker at figuring things out than other kids. Like when my teacher tells us a new way to subtract fractions, it seems obvious to me and not to other kids. But when I'm trying to listen to someone talking or lecturing, my mind starts to wander," she says. Dana describes how she became distracted during a simple discussion about plants during science class:

> It made me think about my garden and what I was going to plant next year. And that made me think about a new kind of chili pepper that I'm going to try to plant for my dad because he likes spicy things. And that made me think about the hot dishes he used to eat when we lived in Singapore. It feels sort of like branches on a tree, and pretty soon I don't know what the discussion is about anymore.[9]

In contrast to those who have predominantly inattentive ADHD, people who have the predominantly hyperactive-impulsive type of ADHD typically find it hard to keep still. They constantly appear restless, fidgeting with their hands and feet or squirming in their chairs. As young children, they might run, jump, and climb constantly. They talk a lot, often interrupting others and speaking out at inappropriate times. In school, they may blurt out the answer to a teacher's question before raising their hands. People with hyperactive-impulsive ADHD often have trouble waiting their turn and may cut in line or simply grab what they want without waiting. They find it hard to stop this constant activity long enough to listen to instructions. And because of their constant movement and impulsive actions, a person with this type of ADHD may have more injuries and accidents than people who do not have the disorder.

Diagnosed with ADHD, fourteen-year-old Zoe Williams from Louisville, Kentucky, is constantly on the move. Her mother, Monnica Williams, describes her daughter as a fireball. "She's the kid in the middle of the dance floor that all the other kids are watching," Williams explains. "And she talks and talks and talks. Sometimes I have to say, 'Zoe, it's not that I don't want to hear what you have to say, but Mom needs a little talking timeout.'"[10]

The third and most common type of ADHD is a combination of the inattentive and hyperactive-impulsive types. People with combined ADHD exhibit symptoms of inattention and hyperactivity equally.

Diagnosing ADHD

Diagnosing ADHD can be difficult. There is no lab test to determine whether a person has the disorder or is simply inattentive and energetic. Moreover, ADHD can be difficult to diagnose because its primary symptoms—inattention and impulsivity—can normally occur in many people. However, although it is normal to have some inattention or impulsivity, these symptoms are more severe and occur more frequently for people with ADHD. Also, in ADHD these symptoms interfere with a person's ability to function normally at school, at work, or in social settings.

To diagnose ADHD, a licensed health care professional, such as a pediatrician, psychologist, or psychiatrist, will conduct a comprehensive evaluation of the patient. The professional will examine the patient to make sure that symptoms are not caused by another medical or psychiatric condition. He or she will interview the patient and review input from parents and teachers to determine the extent of symptoms the patient is experiencing and the

Not Just a Childhood Disorder

For some people, ADHD begins in childhood, and symptoms continue to affect them as adults. For others, new research suggests that ADHD can begin in adults who never showed signs of the disorder as children. In a 2016 study, researchers from the Institute of Psychiatry, Psychology & Neuroscience at King's College London measured more than twenty-two hundred twins for symptoms of childhood ADHD at the ages of five, seven, ten, and twelve. The study participants were also interviewed as young adults at age eighteen to assess ADHD symptoms. The King's College researchers found that nearly 70 percent of young adults with ADHD did not have the disorder in childhood. Also, the participants with adult-onset ADHD reported significant symptoms and impairments. The findings from this study echo similar results from studies in Brazil and New Zealand, which identified a large percentage of adults with ADHD who did not have the disorder as children. "Our research sheds new light on the development and onset of ADHD, but it also brings up many questions about ADHD that arises after childhood," says Louise Arseneault, one of the study's researchers and a professor at King's College London. "How similar or different is 'late-onset' ADHD compared with ADHD that begins in childhood? How and why does late-onset ADHD arise? What treatments are most effective for late-onset ADHD? These are the questions we should now be seeking to answer."

Quoted in King's College London, "ADHD May Emerge After Childhood for Some People, According to New Study," ScienceDaily, May 18, 2016. www.sciencedaily.com.

ways in which those symptoms are impacting his or her life. To receive an ADHD diagnosis, a person under the age of seventeen must exhibit at least six symptoms of the disorder as defined by the *Diagnostic and Statistical Manual of Mental Disorders* of the American Psychiatric Association (APA). For those aged seventeen and older, five symptoms must be present. Symptoms must also be present for at least six months in most areas of the person's life, including home and school. "And, most important, there must be impairment," says Russell A. Barkley, an ADHD expert and clinical professor of psychiatry and pediatrics at the

Medical University of South Carolina in Charleston. "They must be unable to function as well as others—and in fact, are often well below normal—in any of those domains."[11]

Most children are diagnosed with ADHD in elementary school. According to the CDC, the average age of ADHD diagnosis is seven years old. Typically, boys are more likely to be diagnosed with ADHD than girls, at a rate of 13.2 percent compared to 5.6 percent.

The Severity of Symptoms

ADHD affects each person differently. Like those of autism, ADHD symptoms can range from mild to severe. A person with mild symptoms may experience only minor impairment in daily life at school, home, and work. A person with more severe ADHD may experience multiple symptoms, several of which are serious enough to cause significant impairment in the person's daily life.

> "Even when I want to focus, I can't. My mind just wanders. And I'm pretty disorganized and always late. And I've always had a bad memory."[12]
>
> —Sue, a ninth grader with ADHD

As a person ages, the severity of ADHD symptoms can change. Symptoms may lessen or change forms. As symptoms change, children and teens may experience a different type of ADHD as they age. Some adults may continue to experience some of the symptoms of childhood ADHD throughout their life span.

ADHD in Teens

Like children with ADHD, teens with the disorder can be easily distracted and irritable, have trouble concentrating, and experience hyperactivity and lack of impulse control. In addition, the hormonal changes that occur during adolescence may worsen ADHD symptoms.

In teens, symptoms of hyperactivity often include being fidgety or feeling restless. At the same time, inattention and distractibil-

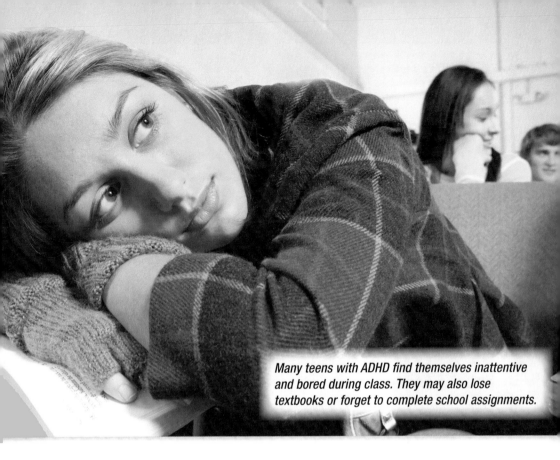

Many teens with ADHD find themselves inattentive and bored during class. They may also lose textbooks or forget to complete school assignments.

ity may become more prominent. Teens may forget assignments at school or lose textbooks. They may become inattentive and bored with classwork. They may interrupt teachers and class-mates. Unable to concentrate for long periods, they may rush through assignments and find it hard to sit still in class. Sue, a ninth grader, says that she has struggled with her grades since middle school. "Even when I want to focus, I can't. My mind just wanders. And I'm pretty disorganized and always late. And I've always had a bad memory,"[12] she says.

Girls and ADHD

ADHD can affect girls differently than boys. Whereas hyperactiv-ity and fidgeting are typical behaviors for boys with ADHD, these symptoms are not always seen in girls with the disorder. For many girls, ADHD presents as the inattentive type. Girls tend to be less disruptive in class than boys and instead have symptoms such as disorganization, distraction, and trouble following directions.

The Puzzle of Focus

One of the more puzzling aspects of ADHD is that people who struggle with chronic symptoms of inattention and focus may have no trouble focusing when they are involved in a particular activity or task. For example, students with ADHD may have trouble paying attention in class or focusing on a homework assignment, but these same teenagers may be able to focus intently and work efficiently when they are playing a sport, painting artwork, doing mechanical tasks, or playing video games. They might not be able to remember facts for the next social studies test, but they can recite statistics about their favorite hockey team. This ability to intently focus on certain activities can be a symptom of ADHD called hyperfocus. Because ADHD causes problems regulating attention on tasks, one task might be hard to concentrate on while another is completely absorbing. At times the focus is so strong that the person becomes oblivious to the world around him or her. "You're focused so intently on something, no other information gets into your brain," says Brandon Ashinoff, a psychologist who studies hyperfocus at the University of Birmingham in England. For people with ADHD, interest is a key factor in hyperfocus. If they love something, they can do it for hours. But if they hate it, they will start, lose focus, and move on to something else. According to hyperfocus researcher Rony Sklar, "It's not about having an attention deficit, it's more a maldistribution of attention. It's not about not being able to concentrate; it's about being able to concentrate in different forms and different intensity."

Quoted in Jenara Nerenberg, "When Adult ADHD Looks Something Like 'Flow,'" *New York Magazine*, July 6, 2016. http://nymag.com.

Also, ADHD symptoms tend to appear at older ages in girls than in boys.

According to some mental health experts, girls often feel more pressure than boys to perform in school and social situations, which leads many to attribute their symptoms of disorganization and forgetfulness to personal flaws. They do not recognize that they have a medical condition that can be treated. Instead, many girls try to fit in with peers by hiding their symptoms. "As an ADHD girl, you're forever falling short of everyone's expectations, never living up to your 'potential.' You try to stay organized, but the lists and notebooks just get lost. You forget plans and goof on names. You struggle to fit in with the other girls, and you feel like everyone else has a cheat sheet of social rules,"[13] says Carolyn Mallon, a nurse who struggled with ADHD as a teen.

Because girls with ADHD show symptoms that are different from those of boys and appear later, these signs have often been missed until very recently. "Girls are not as hyperactive," says Dr. Quinn. "People imagine little boys bouncing off the walls and think: That's what ADHD looks like, and if this girl doesn't look like that then she doesn't have ADHD."[14] As health professionals have learned more about how the disorder presents in girls, however, more girls have been diagnosed with ADHD. Originally, the APA's diagnosis criteria required ADHD symptoms to begin by age seven. But because ADHD symptoms often emerge later in girls, many girls were not diagnosed. In its latest version of the guidelines, the APA has increased the age of symptom onset to twelve, allowing more girls to meet the diagnosis criteria. According to a 2015 study in the *Journal of Clinical Psychiatry*, the number of girls diagnosed with ADHD increased 55 percent between 2003 and 2011 compared to a 40 percent increase for boys.

> "Girls are not as hyperactive. People imagine little boys bouncing off the walls and think: That's what ADHD looks like, and if this girl doesn't look like that then she doesn't have ADHD."[14]
>
> —Dr. Patricia Quinn, director and cofounder of the National Resource Center for Girls and Women with ADHD

Although more girls are being diagnosed with ADHD, many are still being overlooked. Without diagnosis and treatment, girls with ADHD face several psychological risks. Studies show that girls with ADHD can suffer depression, low self-esteem, and anxiety. They may develop eating disorders or start to harm themselves. Struggling to live up to expectations, many girls with ADHD believe that they are simply not smart. "Anxiety and depression turn into low self-esteem and self-loathing, and the risk for self-harm and suicide attempts is four-to-five times that of girls without ADHD,"[15] says Ellen Littman, a clinical psychologist and coauthor of *Understanding Girls with ADHD*. Sometimes the symptoms of depression and anxiety can mask an underlying ADHD disorder. Many girls are misdiagnosed and are treated with antianxiety or depression drugs, which can worsen ADHD symptoms.

Mallon says that her attempts to hide her symptoms made life more difficult in high school:

> I was intelligent enough to leave an impression on my teachers. In fact, I was in the gifted program, but I lacked the organizational skills to meet their academic expectations. If I found a subject interesting, I could do well easily, but if a subject didn't grab me, I could stare at a homework assignment for hours and still not make progress. I would try to follow the class lecture, but if I lost track of what they were discussing, I might as well have wandered alone in the woods. I just couldn't catch up. After a while, I started skipping classes to avoid the shame and embarrassment of having no assignment to turn in or knowing I was going to flunk a test. This contributed to my poor self-image: I felt like a loser and a delinquent. By 11th grade, I wasn't in honors classes at all anymore. I was failing remedial math and getting suspended for truancy. I was drinking, experimenting with drugs, and feeling more miserable than I'd been in my life. This is often the lot of the undiagnosed ADHD girl.[16]

Increasing Diagnosis in Children and Teens

In recent years the number of people diagnosed with ADHD has skyrocketed. A 2015 study published online in the *Journal of Clinical Psychiatry* found that the number of children and teens diagnosed with ADHD increased 43 percent between 2003 and 2011. The study also reported a 52 percent increase in ADHD diagnosis for adolescents between 2003 and 2011. "We found rising rates of ADHD overall and very sharp jumps in certain subgroups," says lead researcher Sean D. Cleary, an associate professor of epidemiology and biostatistics at the Milken Institute School of Public Health at George Washington University. "Parents should be made aware of the findings in case they have a child or teenager that should be evaluated for the disorder, which can persist into adulthood." The study did not look at the reasons behind the increasing number of diagnoses. "Additional studies must be done to identify the underlying cause of the increase,"[17] Cleary says.

Many people believe that wider awareness about ADHD has led to more children and teens being identified as having the disorder instead of slipping through the cracks. Growing demands on students, particularly in high school, have also led to an increase in diagnosis. Quyen Epstein-Ngo, a psychology researcher at the University of Michigan, is not surprised by the rising diagnosis rate and points out that it is consistent with trends that US health professionals have been noticing for years. "It could be that the last several years have seen an increased ability, or willingness, to recognize that older adolescents who are still struggling could require more formal help and support," he says. "Alternatively, it could be that increased pressures on adolescents to perform and achieve are leading to a push for more ADHD assessments."[18] Michael Manos,

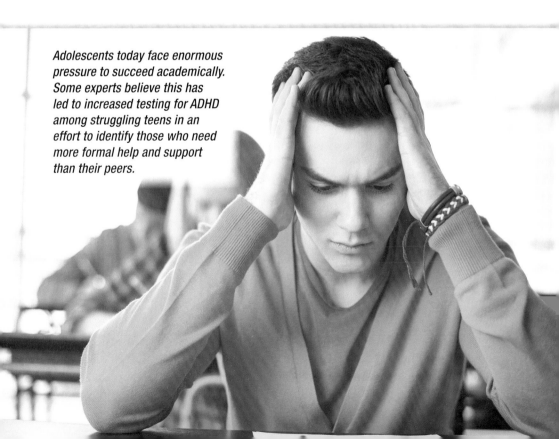

Adolescents today face enormous pressure to succeed academically. Some experts believe this has led to increased testing for ADHD among struggling teens in an effort to identify those who need more formal help and support than their peers.

the head of the Center for Pediatric Behavioral Health at Cleveland Clinic Children's Hospital, agrees. "Almost essentially, it's associated with a child's ability to manage themselves in school," he says. "We now have placed such an emphasis on academic success as being almost critical; it's no longer good enough for a child to have a high IQ and good grades. They have to have great grades. So you have an increase in the prevalence of ADHD in adolescents primarily because we're recognizing a less than optimal response."[19]

Not a Perfect Diagnosis

Although increasing awareness about the disorder and its symptoms has helped many people receive an accurate diagnosis, there is no foolproof test to determine if a person has ADHD. Diagnosing ADHD is a subjective process based on the evaluation of a health professional who relies on input from parents and teachers. "In one of the most widely used and well-validated diagnostic tests, a child needs to demonstrate 6 of 9 specific behaviors on a standardized form to be diagnosed, and thereby qualify for disability accommodations. But the assessments, usually completed by a teacher and parent, are subjective. They must decide, for example, whether a child 'often' has 'difficulty organizing tasks and activities'—or 'very often,'"[20] says Dimitri Christakis, director of the Center for Child Health, Behavior, and Development at Seattle Children's Research Institute.

Because diagnosing ADHD is a subjective process, some people are concerned that ADHD is being overdiagnosed. "Having spent about 25 years in education, I have seen teachers quickly assume that students who are more active than their classmates (and who are more active than their teachers' tolerance for high activity levels) require medication. The rush to saddle them with a disorder, with little prior intervention, contributes to misidentification and societal over-medication," says Donna Ford, a professor of education and human development at Vanderbilt University. "There are several problems that contribute to ADHD misdiagnosis. The first is the subjective and limited nature of the evaluations used to diagnose an already high-energy population (kids). A checklist of behaviors should not be the only or primary source of an evaluation when so much is at stake. Observation over a period of time and in multiple settings are needed,"[21] she says.

In addition, the scarcity of child psychiatrists in the United States means that diagnosing ADHD often falls to pediatricians and family doctors, many of whom are not adequately trained to do so. "When I trained, most of pediatrics was treating infectious disease," says William Wittert, a fifty-seven-year-old pediatrician in Libertyville, Illinois. "But we don't treat bacterial meningitis anymore. We are being asked to evaluate and handle mental health issues in kids like ADHD. We have to get up to speed." Dr. Wittert describes the imprecise nature of his evaluation process, saying he would review a list of vague symptoms such as distractibility and forgetfulness with the patient. "If you had enough yesses, then you pretty much got the diagnosis of ADHD,"[22] he says. In New York, Harriet Hellman, a certified pediatric nurse practitioner who is licensed to make mental health diagnoses, agrees that the process is often inexact. Hellman says sometimes she would diagnose patients with the disorder through instinct, a "hair-on-the-back-of-your-neck feeling."[23]

> "There are several problems that contribute to ADHD misdiagnosis. The first is the subjective and limited nature of the evaluations used to diagnose an already high-energy population (kids)."[21]
>
> —Donna Ford, a professor of education and human development at Vanderbilt University

Increased Awareness Aids Achievement

Before requesting an evaluation for ADHD, families should make sure that the pediatrician or health professional is trained to diagnose and treat ADHD and feels competent to do so. After a diagnosis, families should discuss with the health professional the reasons underlying the diagnosis and possible treatment approaches. Experts in ADHD also recommend getting a second opinion from a mental health specialist if possible. Although the process of diagnosing ADHD may not be perfect in many ways, the increased awareness of the disorder and its symptoms has helped many children and teens achieve their potential.

CHAPTER TWO

What Causes ADHD?

Although many scientists have studied ADHD, researchers do not fully understand the disorder and have not yet determined its exact cause. Many scientists believe that there is no single cause of ADHD. Instead, they believe several different factors could increase a person's likelihood of developing ADHD, including genetic, biological, and environmental factors.

Having one of these risk factors does not mean the person will definitely develop ADHD; it means only that the person has a statistically greater chance of developing it than someone without such a risk factor. Awareness of risk factors for ADHD can help a person determine if he or she is at risk of developing the disorder. Armed with this knowledge, the person will be better able to recognize any symptoms that might appear and seek diagnosis and treatment for them as early as possible.

Genetic Links

Although the exact causes of ADHD are unknown, scientists believe that heredity is a major factor in determining who develops ADHD. Several studies on ADHD have shown that the disorder runs in families; a person with a parent or sibling with ADHD has a higher chance of developing the disorder than someone who does not. According to the American Academy of Child and Adolescent Psychiatry, about 25 percent of children with ADHD have a parent who has ADHD, and 30 percent have or will have a sibling with ADHD.

To understand the genetic influences on ADHD, researchers have studied identical twins. They found that when one twin develops ADHD, the other twin has an 80 percent chance of developing the disorder as well. Because identical twins have the same genes, researchers believe that these results suggest a strong genetic component to ADHD. However, because the twins did not both develop ADHD in all cases, researchers believe that ADHD is not caused by one gene but rather by a combination of many genes and environmental factors.

A number of studies have identified two genes, DRD4 and DAT1, that are involved with the neurotransmitter dopamine and may play a role in ADHD. Neurotransmitters are chemicals that send signals across synapses—gaps between the brain's nerve cells—and affect how a person feels, thinks, and behaves. In people with ADHD, a longer version of the DRD4 gene may make their nerve cells less sensitive to normal amounts of dopamine. As a result, they need more dopamine to activate the cells. Risk taking,

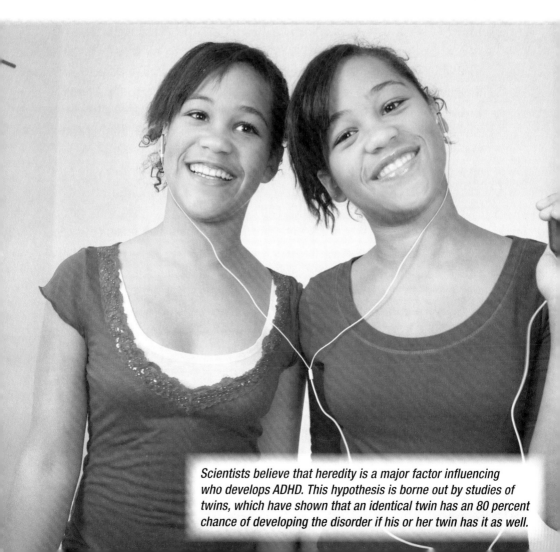

Scientists believe that heredity is a major factor influencing who develops ADHD. This hypothesis is borne out by studies of twins, which have shown that an identical twin has an 80 percent chance of developing the disorder if his or her twin has it as well.

impulsiveness, and restless behavior can stimulate the brain and trigger the release of dopamine. The DAT1 gene may help regulate dopamine activity in the brain by affecting how quickly the neurotransmitter is absorbed from the synapse. Some people with ADHD have also been found to have a longer version of the DAT1 gene than people without the disorder.

Ongoing research continues to uncover additional genetic links to ADHD. At the National Human Genome Research Institute (NHGRI), an international team of researchers working on a genetic study of ADHD have identified a gene associated with the disorder called LPHN3. The LPHN3 gene is involved in neuron signaling in the area of the brain related to behavioral response. The researchers screened the DNA of 6,360 people, half of whom had ADHD, which enabled them to identify a specific region of the LPHN3 gene that was linked to ADHD symptoms. Fine mapping of the DNA of the gene allowed researchers to pinpoint variants in the DNA code that may affect the gene's function and trigger ADHD. "Our efforts revealed important functional sequences within the *LPHN3* gene that may be important in neurologic health," says senior author Maximilian Muenke, chief of the NHGRI's Medical Genetics Branch. "This study is a critical step to better understanding this disease and creates a new opportunity for developing novel and more personalized treatments for patients."[24]

In 2016 researchers at the Massachusetts Institute of Technology (MIT) and New York University linked ADHD to another gene mutation that produces a defect in the brain's thalamic reticular nucleus (TRN), an area that is responsible for blocking out distracting sensory input. The TRN acts as a gatekeeper and prevents unnecessary information from being sent on to the brain areas where thought and planning happen. "We receive all kinds of information from different sensory regions, and it all goes into the thalamus," says Guoping Feng, a professor of neuroscience at MIT and a senior author of the study. "All this information has to be filtered. Not everything we sense goes through."[25] If the TRN gatekeeper does not work properly, too much information passes through it. This overload of information can cause a person to become easily distracted or overwhelmed and can cause attention and learning problems.

What Does Not Cause ADHD

Over the years several theories have emerged about what causes ADHD. Some people believe that ADHD is triggered by consuming the chemical additives in food or eating too much sugar. Others claim that poor parenting or allowing a child to watch too much television is the cause of ADHD symptoms. ADHD experts stress that these theories have little scientific evidence to back them up.

In the case of sugar, several studies have not been able to prove that consuming sugar affects a child's behavior or cognitive skills. Some parents and teachers still insist that consuming sugar does cause children to become more hyperactive and increases ADHD symptoms. The explanation, however, may rest more with the parent or teacher than with the child. Researchers studied the interaction of parents and children when some parents were told that their child was given a dose of sugar and others were told their child received a nonsugar placebo. In reality, all of the children received the placebo. But the parents who believed their child had consumed the sugar were more likely to rate the child's behavior as more hyperactive and were quicker to criticize their children.

The researchers studied a gene called PTCHD1 and found that the loss of this gene most affects the TRN area of the brain. They also found that a mutation in the PTCHD1 gene caused hyperactivity and attention-deficit symptoms in mice. This gene mutation may have caused these symptoms by affecting the channels that carry potassium ions to the brain and preventing the TRN neurons from inhibiting the thalamus's signals. According to Joshua Gordon, an associate professor of psychiatry at Columbia University,

> The authors convincingly demonstrate that specific behavioral consequences of the PTCHD1 mutation—attention and sleep—arise from an alteration of a specific protein in a specific brain region, the thalamic reticular nucleus. These findings provide a clear and straightforward pathway from gene to behavior and suggest a pathway toward novel treatments for neurodevelopmental disorders.[26]

Researchers suspect that ADHD is not caused by a single genetic defect. Instead, they believe that the disorder results from many genes working together. When some of those genes contain mutations, the body and brain's systems that control behavior and attention are disrupted. "This is one of the most exciting and most rapidly developing areas of research in ADHD at this time," says Russell A. Barkley. "What all this means is that ADHD is caused by multiple genes. Each gene makes a relatively small contribution to the risk for having the disorder. But a child who gets enough of those ADHD-risk genes will manifest symptoms severe enough to be diagnosed with the disorder."[27]

Brain Structure and Connections

Because the human brain controls basic body functions, movements, thoughts, and emotions, factors that affect its structure, connections, and activity may play a role in ADHD. Brain imaging studies have revealed significant differences in the brains of children with ADHD compared to children without the disorder. Several studies using advanced imaging have found a size difference in certain parts of the brain in people with ADHD. These areas include the cerebellum, prefrontal cortex, caudate nucleus, and the frontal and temporal lobes. Other studies have shown that children with ADHD have overall smaller brain volume than children without the disorder.

In a 2011 study, researchers at the Kennedy Krieger Institute in Baltimore found that preschool children with ADHD symptoms had a significantly smaller caudate nucleus. The caudate nucleus is a brain structure in the subcortical region that plays an important role in cognitive function and motor control.

> "What all this means is that ADHD is caused by multiple genes. Each gene makes a relatively small contribution to the risk for having the disorder. But a child who gets enough of those ADHD-risk genes will manifest symptoms severe enough to be diagnosed with the disorder."[27]
>
> —Russell A. Barkley, a leading expert on ADHD and a professor of psychiatry and pediatrics at the Medical University of South Carolina in Charleston

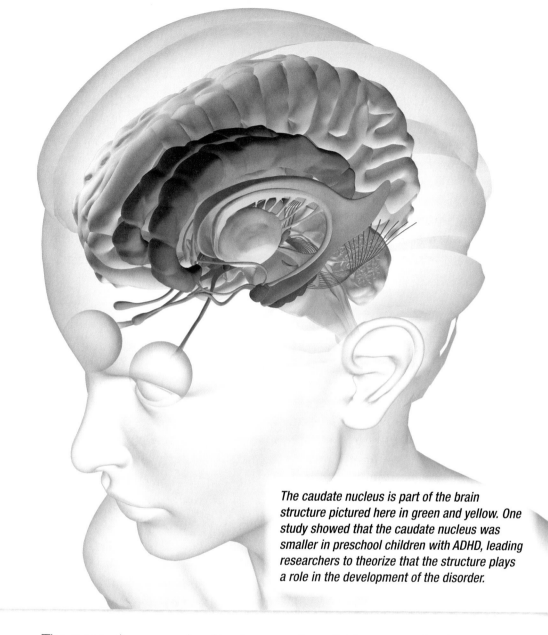

The caudate nucleus is part of the brain structure pictured here in green and yellow. One study showed that the caudate nucleus was smaller in preschool children with ADHD, leading researchers to theorize that the structure plays a role in the development of the disorder.

The researchers examined brain scans from thirteen preschoolers with ADHD symptoms of attention problems and impulsivity and thirteen children without these symptoms. They found that the children with ADHD symptoms had a smaller caudate nucleus. Moreover, the smaller this area of the brain was, the greater the level of symptoms that the child's parents reported. The researchers concluded that differences in brain development, particularly in the caudate nucleus, were a significant factor in children who showed early symptoms of ADHD. "Clinically, this abnormal brain development sets the stage for the symptoms of ADHD that contribute to cognitive challenges and problems in school," says lead author Mark Mahone, director of neuropsychology at Kennedy Krieger. The researchers hope that their findings may help doctors develop better treatments for patients with ADHD. "Earlier identification and treatment of children presenting with attention problems in the preschool years may minimize the impact of ADHD in the long-term,"[28] Mahone says.

Differences in brain structure may not change as a child matures into an adolescent and an adult. The lasting differences may explain why ADHD symptoms persist for some people into adulthood. In 2015 researchers at the University of Cambridge in England used magnetic resonance imaging to study the brain and memory function in young adults. They found that the volunteers with ADHD had reduced brain volume in the caudate nucleus. Memory tests also showed that the young adults with ADHD had poorer memory function compared to those without ADHD. One in three ADHD subjects failed the memory test compared to less than one in twenty without the disorder. For those who passed the memory test, participants with ADHD scored an average of 6 percent lower than the other volunteers. The researchers believe that these results demonstrate that differences in brain structure related to ADHD, particularly the caudate nucleus, can persist into adulthood and continue to cause problems for young adults. "In the controls, when the test got harder, the caudate nucleus went up a gear in its activity, and this is likely to have helped solve the memory problems," says study author Dr. Graham Murray. "But in the group with adolescent ADHD, this region of the brain is smaller and doesn't seem to be able to respond to increasing memory demands with the results that memory performance suffers."[29]

> "This abnormal brain development sets the stage for the symptoms of ADHD that contribute to cognitive challenges and problems in school."[28]
>
> —Mark Mahone, director of neuropsychology at the Kennedy Krieger Institute

Some studies have found that the brains of people with ADHD not only possess a different structure from those of people without the disorder, but they also function differently. These studies have shown less activity in the brain's frontal lobes in people with ADHD than in others. This region of the brain is responsible for executive functions such as thinking, paying attention, and planning. These areas inhibit behavior and help a person envision potential consequences before acting. The less active these inhibiting areas of the brain are, the more likely a person will have difficulty maintaining self-control. Weak connections between areas in the frontal lobes may be another factor in ADHD.

Chemical Imbalances

Brain chemistry may also play a role in ADHD. Research suggests that people with ADHD have neurotransmitter imbalances. These imbalances can cause the message from the brain to the body to get mixed up or not delivered. When this happens, ADHD symptoms may occur.

In addition to dopamine, another neurotransmitter linked to ADHD is norepinephrine. An imbalance in the levels of dopamine and norepinephrine has been found in the brains of people with ADHD compared to people without the disorder. Both of these neurotransmitters influence a person's impulsive behavior and help regulate emotional responses, but dopamine also affects attention. In several studies, scientists have found that lower levels of dopamine are associated with ADHD symptoms. In addition, the brain scans of ADHD patients revealed that they had significantly fewer dopamine receptors in their reward circuits than healthy people, which would reduce the brain's ability to receive dopamine. The lower the number of dopamine receptors that exist, the greater the person's symptoms and inattention.

Other studies are examining the role of another neurotransmitter called gamma-aminobutyric acid (GABA) in ADHD. GABA helps to regulate communication between brain cells and acts as an inhibitory chemical to reduce the activity of neurons. GABA influences behavior, cognition, and the body's response to stress. In a 2012 study, researchers from the Kennedy Krieger Institute

Being Born Late and ADHD

Babies born late may have a higher risk of developing ADHD. A 2012 study by researchers in the Netherlands showed that babies born after a forty-two-week pregnancy had a higher risk of developing behavioral problems than babies born at term, between thirty-nine and forty-one weeks. In the study, researchers followed more than five thousand babies and had the babies' parents fill out a questionnaire when the children reached the ages of eighteen months and thirty-six months. The questionnaire asked about the child's behavior and is commonly used to identify ADHD and other developmental and emotional problems. The researchers found that post-term babies were more than 2.5 times as likely to have ADHD at these ages than babies born at term. "Post-term children have a considerably higher risk of clinically relevant problem behavior and are more than twice as likely as term born children to have clinical ADHD," says the study's lead author, Hanan El Marroun. "Further research is needed in order to determine the causes of post-term birth and to minimize the long-term consequences. It is also important that further research is carried out to demonstrate a causal relation between post-term birth and behavioral problems and longer follow-ups would also be advantageous."

Quoted in Rebecca Smith, "Overdue Babies More Likely to Have ADHD: Research," *Telegraph*, May 3, 2012. www.telegraph.co.uk.

and Cincinnati Children's Hospital Medical Center found significantly lower concentrations of GABA in the brains of children with ADHD compared to children without the diagnosis.

Environmental Factors

Environmental factors may interact with genes to contribute to ADHD symptoms. Changes in brain structure, function, and chemistry may be caused by genetics, but they may also be caused by environmental factors. Some research studies suggest that childhood exposure to certain environmental factors may affect the early development of the brain, which can lead to ADHD symptoms. These factors include substances consumed during pregnancy, secondhand smoke, lead, and other toxins.

The substances used by the mother during pregnancy may cause changes in brain development in the unborn child that may be a factor in ADHD. "Fetuses exposed to alcohol can develop fetal alcohol effects or fetal alcohol syndrome, and the prominent features for both are the symptoms you see in ADHD,"[30] says Dr. Mark L. Wolraich, chief of developmental and behavioral pediatrics at the University of Oklahoma Health Sciences Center. Studies also suggest a possible connection between a pregnant woman's cigarette smoking and ADHD in her child. A 2014 study also suggested that use of nicotine patches and gum while pregnant may be linked to ADHD in the unborn child. "We've been lulled into a false sense of security, thinking that if we can just get mothers to stop smoking and onto nicotine replacement, it will protect against any kinds of fetal damage in the developing child. This is a stark injection of reality about how that may not be the case,"[31] says Dr. Timothy Wilens, director of the Center for Addiction Medicine and acting chief of child psychiatry at Massachusetts General Hospital in Boston.

> "Fetuses exposed to alcohol can develop fetal alcohol effects or fetal alcohol syndrome, and the prominent features for both are the symptoms you see in ADHD."[30]
>
> —Dr. Mark L. Wolraich, chief of developmental and behavioral pediatrics at the University of Oklahoma Health Sciences Center

After a child is born, exposure to secondhand smoke may increase the risk of ADHD. According to a 2015 study by researchers in Spain, children exposed to cigarette smoke at home for as little as one hour a day are up to three times more likely to have ADHD compared to children from smoke-free homes. The link was stronger for children who were exposed to one or more hours of secondhand smoke daily. "The association between secondhand smoke and global mental problems was mostly due to the impact of secondhand smoke on the attention-deficit and hyperactivity disorder,"[32] explain the study's authors.

Exposure to high levels of lead as a young child may be another factor in ADHD. Lead can be found in plumbing fixtures and paint in older buildings. In a 2016 study, researchers found that exposure to

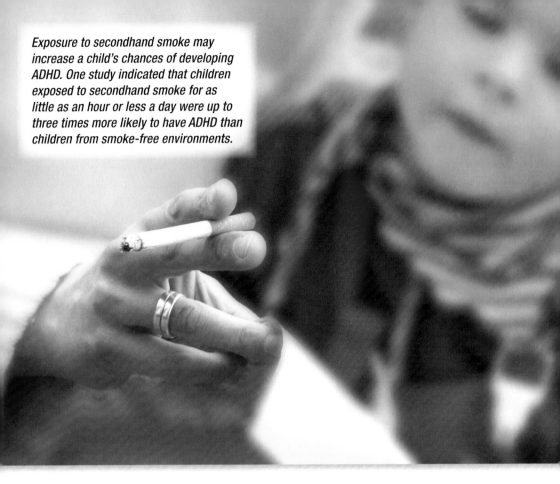

Exposure to secondhand smoke may increase a child's chances of developing ADHD. One study indicated that children exposed to secondhand smoke for as little as an hour or less a day were up to three times more likely to have ADHD than children from smoke-free environments.

even small amounts of lead can contribute to ADHD symptoms in children with a specific HFE C282Y gene mutation. The researchers measured blood lead level in healthy children ages six to seventeen. Half of the children were diagnosed with ADHD, but the other half were not. The researchers found an increased association with lead exposure and ADHD symptoms in participants who had the gene mutation. Increased lead exposure also increased ADHD symptoms in children without the gene mutation, but not as consistently. The study reveals important information about how environmental factors, while not causing ADHD, can nonetheless influence ADHD symptoms. "This research is valuable to the scientific community as it bridges genetic and environmental factors and helps to illustrate one possible route to ADHD. Further, it demonstrates the potential to ultimately prevent conditions like ADHD by understanding how genes and environmental exposures combine,"[33] says lead researcher Joel Nigg, a professor of psychiatry and behavioral neuroscience at the Oregon Health Science and University School of Medicine.

Premature Birth and Low Birth Weight

Babies who are born prematurely and have a very low birth weight may have a higher risk of developing several mental disorders as adults, including depression, ADHD, and anxiety, compared to babies born at a healthy weight. According to the CDC, about 8 percent of babies born in the United States had a low birth weight of less than 5.5 pounds (2.5 kg) in 2013, and about 1.4 percent of babies had a birth weight of less than 3.3 pounds (1.5 kg). The majority of these babies—70 percent—were born prematurely.

In a 2015 study, researchers examined eighty-four adults who were born at an extremely low birth weight and compared them to ninety adults who were born at a normal weight. They assessed each participant for psychiatric disorders. The participants who were born at an extremely low weight were 2.5 times more likely to develop a psychiatric disorder as an adult than those participants who had a normal birth weight. Also, the participants whose mothers presented symptoms of premature labor and received steroid treatment during pregnancy, used to improve a premature baby's lung function, were almost 4.5 times more likely to develop a psychiatric disorder compared to normal-birth-weight participants. "Importantly, we have identified psychiatric risks that may develop for extremely low-birth-weight survivors as they become adults, and this understanding will help us better predict, detect and treat mental disorders in this population,"[34] says the research team leader, Ryan Van Lieshout, a professor of psychiatry and neurosciences at McMaster University in Canada.

Brain Injury

In some cases, an injury to the brain may increase a person's risk for ADHD. In a 2015 study published in the journal *Pediatrics*, researchers found that children who have suffered a brain injury are more likely to have problems with attention than children who have not. Moreover, these problems may not develop immediately; instead, they could surface months after the injury. Study author March Kongs, a doctoral candidate at VU University Amsterdam, says that the attention problems were "very short lapses in focus, causing children to be slower."[35] Kongs's team examined more than one hundred children ages six to thirteen who had experienced a traumatic brain injury (TBI). These injuries ranged in severity from a concussion that resulted in a headache or vomiting to a head injury that caused the child to lose consciousness for more than thirty minutes. The team compared the TBI children to a group of children who had experienced a non-head trauma. Approximately eighteen months after the children's accidents, their parents and teachers rated their attention and other health measures. The team discovered that the TBI children had more lapses in attention and slower processing speeds, along with other issues such as anxiety. Although a TBI may increase the risk of ADHD, it is considered a minor risk factor because only a small number of children with ADHD have suffered this kind of injury.

The increased risk of ADHD after a TBI also extends into adulthood. In 2015 a Canadian study published in the *Journal of Psychiatric Research* found a link between TBI and a history of ADHD in adults. The researchers surveyed nearly four thousand adults aged eighteen and older and defined TBI as having a trauma to the head that resulted in either a loss of consciousness for at least five minutes or required an overnight stay in a hospital. The researchers found that 5.9 percent of participants with a history of TBI reported having been diagnosed with ADHD, and another 6.6 percent screened positive for ADHD during the survey. "These new data suggest a significant association between ADHD and TBI," says one of the principal investigators, Robert Mann. "We see that adults with TBI are more than twice as likely than those without to report symptoms of ADHD."[36] Some experts believe that this occurs because a TBI causes changes in the brain that increase the risk of ADHD developing. Other scientists point out that it may be the opposite—having ADHD could increase a person's risk of falling or having an accident that results in a TBI. More studies are needed to better understand the link between ADHD and TBI and how it affects the development and treatment of each.

A Combination of Factors

Some illnesses have a medical cause that is easy to identify and treat. A person with strep throat takes antibiotics. People with high cholesterol manage their disease with diet and medication. ADHD, however, is more complicated. It does not appear to be caused by a single factor and cannot be cured with a pill. Instead, ADHD may be caused by a combination of several factors. Although scientists do not understand the exact cause of ADHD, knowing the potential factors can make it easier to identify the disorder earlier and seek treatment. According to Barkley,

> We have much more to learn about ADHD and its potential causes. Nevertheless, great advances have been made in . . . understanding the possible causes of ADHD. All of the evidence to date points to genetically based neurological factors as being the most important in explaining the extent of ADHD in the population. A smaller percentage of cases of ADHD appear to be due to acquired injuries to the developing brain, such as through toxins consumed by the mother during pregnancy or child after birth. When we fully comprehend what causes this disorder, perhaps we will also discover how to cure it.[37]

CHAPTER THREE

What Is It Like to Live with ADHD?

Grace Friedman knew something was wrong in fourth grade. She paid attention in class but had trouble remembering what she learned. She spent twice as long as her classmates to complete assignments. When she was diagnosed at age eleven with ADHD, Friedman felt relieved to have a name for what she was experiencing. "It was a great relief to know why I was struggling, but having an ADHD diagnosis did not in and of itself resolve any of my challenges, it simply categorized and in some cases amplified them. As I soon learned, like most, I was prescribed some meds and then left to my own devices to understand, manage and adapt to my 'disorder,'" she says. Friedman describes ADHD as an invisible disorder, which makes it difficult to explain how it feels to those who have not experienced it. She likens living with ADHD to a race:

> Envision this: five teens line up to race the 1000 meters. Four of them wear shorts and sneakers, and the fifth is wearing a hazmat suit and a 30-pound [14 kg] backpack. It should not surprise anyone that the fifth runner will not likely outpace the others. Now imagine the hazmat suit and the 30-pound backpack are transparent—that is what it is like to have ADHD. Teens with ADHD often feel ashamed, stigmatized, embarrassed and isolated. Everyone wonders why we are not the fastest runner.[38]

Friedman has become an advocate to help others like herself, writing an online guide and creating a website for teens with ADHD. "I am a runner with the backpack, and I know I may never outpace my peers, but I have to run anyway—life requires it," she says. "I could choose to give up or I can race knowing that I may not always win, but will certainly lose if I do not try. I choose to race."[39]

A High Social Cost

For children with ADHD, life can be a flurry of activity. Many ADHD children run and climb excessively. For those around them, it seems as if the child is being driven by a motor that never shuts off. And although these children can be very sociable, their hyperactive and impulsive behavior can cause problems at school, at home, and on the playground. Often they are unable to stop moving or even stop talking. Too impatient to wait their turn, they interrupt others, cut in line, and grab the toy they want. They are easily frustrated, and their emotions can erupt like a volcano, causing them to lash out violently at those around them or have a temper tantrum. Often this behavior causes them to act younger and more immaturely than their peers. It can also have a high social cost, creating problems in their relationships with family, friends, and teachers.

> "It was a great relief to know why I was struggling, but having an ADHD diagnosis did not in and of itself resolve any of my challenges, it simply categorized and in some cases amplified them."[38]
>
> —Grace Friedman, a teen with ADHD

Kerri Meenagh's ten-year-old daughter, Saorla, is a boundless ball of energy who rarely sits still. Her mother worries that her ADHD symptoms may make it more difficult for Saorla to make friends. "Saorla is such a good kid, such an empathetic kid, but if she's tired, she becomes 'Hurricane Saorla,'" says Meenagh. Like a younger child, Saorla often has difficulty transitioning from one activity to another. During a class trip to the zoo, for example, Saorla resisted moving from one exhibit to the next with the rest of her classmates. She threw a huge temper tantrum, complete with kicking and screaming, as her mother pulled her away. Meenagh

Negative Impact of ADHD on Everyday Life

ADHD can impact a young person's life at home and at school. It can put stress on relationships with family, friends, teachers, and others. In a European survey, almost half of parents and caregivers of youth with ADHD reported negative impacts on school life for those kids. Nearly one in three participants reported that life at home was also negatively impacted by ADHD.

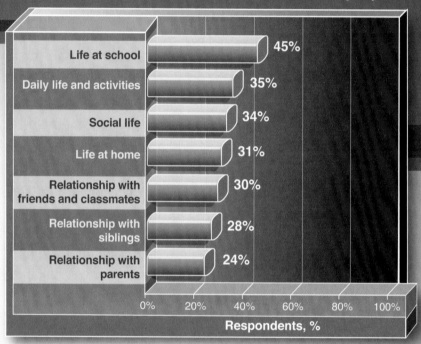

Perceived Negative Impact of ADHD on Everyday Life

Category	Percentage
Life at school	45%
Daily life and activities	35%
Social life	34%
Life at home	31%
Relationship with friends and classmates	30%
Relationship with siblings	28%
Relationship with parents	24%

Respondents, %

Source: ADHD Institute, "Impact of ADHD." www.adhd-institute.com.

says that Saorla's tantrums can often last for an hour. "I was very aware that everyone was looking at us," she says. "I was mortified, but mainly I was scared that she was going to be labeled by the other parents as a kid other kids shouldn't be friends with." Because Saorla acts with the maturity of a younger child, her friends are often younger children rather than her same-aged classmates. "She operates more at a seven-year-old level, so her friends tend to be younger," says Meenagh. "She can be very silly—silly to the point that her classmates say she's too silly for them."[40]

Difficulty in School

As children with ADHD grow into teens, their hyperactivity tends to decrease or show as restlessness and fidgeting. As teens, they might struggle more with attention and impulsivity. At the same time, the expectations teens face, both at school and in social circles, greatly increase. Typical teens are expected to be able to handle a growing number of decisions on their own. When moving from elementary and middle school to high school, teens receive less structure and teacher oversight in their classes and are expected to be responsible for following along and keeping up with classmates. These expectations can cause many difficulties for teens with ADHD. Dr. Thomas E. Brown, an international expert on ADHD, explains:

> In the transition into middle school or junior high school, most early adolescents are confronted not only with escalating academic demands in class and in homework requirements but also with a much more complex daily environment, with multiple teachers, increased need to organize materials and keep track of multiple assignments, hourly changes from one group and classroom to another, and expectations of more independent functioning with less intensive supervision from teachers and parents. Research has shown that the transition into middle school tends to be especially disruptive for children with ADHD. Although many show some gradual decline in their ADHD symptoms during middle to later childhood, the transition to middle school tends to disrupt that decline significantly and to cause increased impairment of functioning.[41]

Without support, teens with ADHD often have lower grades in school and lower scores on standardized tests. Struggling to manage distractibility and poor concentration, these teens may forget assignments or lose textbooks. Some may have trouble paying attention in class, but others may become excessively attentive and interrupt teachers and classmates. They may rush through assignments, scoring poorly because they did not read

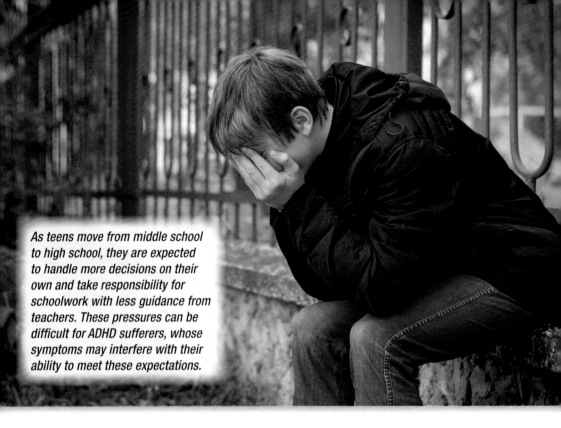

As teens move from middle school to high school, they are expected to handle more decisions on their own and take responsibility for schoolwork with less guidance from teachers. These pressures can be difficult for ADHD sufferers, whose symptoms may interfere with their ability to meet these expectations.

the directions completely. They may also find it hard to sit still during class. All of these behaviors can add up to bad grades, which can lead to failing classes. In addition, disruptive behaviors can get students in trouble with teachers and administrators.

Fourteen-year-old Ali Comstock was diagnosed with ADHD at age five. When she started middle school, her classwork became more demanding. By eighth grade she was barely making a C average in her classes and was becoming increasingly anxious about being unprepared for class. "Whenever I got back a test with a low score, it bummed me out for the whole day. I could never enjoy myself because I was constantly worried about school. Even when I'd go to bed, I'd lie there for a long time thinking about the homework that I didn't finish or the project that I hadn't even started,"[42] she says.

Ali's parents noticed her struggles. "For a while, I was worried that she was going to flunk out of eighth grade because she couldn't juggle assignments," says Ali's mother, Kathleen Comstock. "Getting organized was a problem for her. Finding important papers or her assignment pad became almost an impossible task for her. She wasn't turning in her work on time. Many times I'd find out that Ali had a big project due the next day and that she'd never mentioned it to me or started it."[43]

Ali's parents decided to get their daughter help. The summer before ninth grade, Ali met weekly with an ADHD coach who worked with her to develop strategies for dealing with her ADHD in school. One of the problems they tackled was enabling her to be better organized so she could remember her assignments. Ali often did not write down her assignments because she thought she could remember them without doing so. Or if she did write them down, she misplaced her notes. "Dee [her ADHD coach] taught me strategies that gave me more control. Now I write my assignments on individual sheets of paper and keep them in a folder," Ali says.

> When I get home I take a short break; then I take out my homework folder. I look through each assignment and get started on the hardest subjects, like math and science. As I finish each assignment, I move it from the "to-do" side of the folder to the "completed" side, so I can see what I've accomplished. At first, I'd take a break after I finished each subject and be finished around dinnertime. But now I don't even need breaks, and I'm usually finished by four-thirty![44]

The Effect on Relationships

In addition to causing difficulties in school, ADHD can also have an impact on a person's relationships with family, friends, and classmates. Research shows that children and teens with ADHD often have fewer friendships and are more likely to be ignored or rejected by peers than children without the disorder. They are also more likely to be involved in bullying—either as a victim or a bully.

ADHD symptoms may cause a person to behave in ways that irritate others. People with ADHD may interrupt friends and classmates and have trouble filtering their comments. They can be intense and demanding and have trouble waiting their turn. In a conversation, they may become distracted and lose focus, causing them to appear as if they are not listening and to misunderstand what the other person is saying. Some people, especially children, with ADHD struggle with self-control and may have physical outbursts or temper tantrums when it is no longer age-appropriate. Many people with ADHD do not even realize that these behaviors are causing a problem with their relationships with family and friends.

Lisa Aro's daughter sometimes has problems filtering her comments and can be very blunt when interacting with others at school. "We were at an awards assembly honoring my daughter and her project partner for a community service learning project where they made colorful pillowcases for a battered women's shelter," Aro recalls. "The principal congratulated her and joked, 'Those are some great pillowcases, you should make me one.' My daughter looked at him blankly and said, 'You have a job, you have money, you can buy your own pillowcase.'" Aro explained to her daughter that her comments were not the best way to handle the situation. In response, her daughter "slumped her shoulders, let out a truly exasperated sigh, and said, 'Is there a book on social skills? Because I really need one.'"[45]

ADHD symptoms can cause stress at home as well as in school. When teens with ADHD procrastinate or are disorganized and distracted when doing homework or household chores, it can lead to conflict with parents. Kathleen Comstock admits that fights over homework created stress at home for both her and her daughter. "I resented the amount of time I had to spend with her on homework," says Comstock.

I work full-time and hated coming home and having to work with her for an hour on a math assignment that should have taken 15 minutes. She couldn't focus and got up from the table every five minutes for a glass of water, something to eat, or to answer the phone. We started arguing about homework all the time. Yelling didn't solve anything, though. Ali sat there and didn't say anything, and I felt bad for yelling. I tried to figure out what part of her behavior was due to ADHD and what part was simply being a teenager.[46]

ADHD and Working Memory

Many people with ADHD experience problems with their working memory function. Although they can recite the lyrics of an entire song or quote from a movie they saw years ago, they cannot seem to remember the directions that a teacher gave the class five minutes earlier. They can read and understand an entire page of text, but only a few minutes later they cannot remember what they have read. Working memory stores a small amount of information so that it can be used for a few seconds. For example, to do mental math, a person must read or hear the numbers, hold them in working memory, and add them to find the answer. Working memory has an important role in concentration and following directions. People with working memory problems can have trouble remembering what comes next in a set of instructions. A student may have trouble remembering what sentence to write while also trying to remember how to spell the words. Working memory also helps students remember what items they need to pay attention to while completing a task. Therefore, kids with weak working memory skills may find it hard to focus on a task and have trouble remembering the steps required to complete the task.

Regulating Emotions

Everyone experiences a variety of emotions—from frustration and fear to pride and excitement—every day. For people with ADHD, managing and responding to this array of emotions can be challenging. "Many people with ADHD tend to get quickly flooded with frustration, enthusiasm, anger, affection, worry, boredom, discouragement, or other emotions," says Brown.

> They may vent their momentary anger on a friend or family member with hurtful intensity that does not take into account that this is a person whom they love and do not want to hurt. People with ADHD report that momentary emotion often gobbles up all the space in their head, as a computer virus can gobble up all the space on a hard drive, crowding out other important feelings and thoughts.[47]

Life during the teenage years is an emotional roller coaster for almost everyone, but for teens with ADHD who already struggle with regulating their emotions, it can be especially challenging. For example, a teen with ADHD may become overwhelmed by emotions and fly into a rage when a parent does not let him or her use the car to go out with friends. Although many teens might argue or complain in this situation, a teen with ADHD may escalate into throwing objects or punching a wall. "A teen without ADHD might momentarily consider such extreme responses, but usually would inhibit them because he is able to keep in mind, despite the momentary intensity of anger, that this is a parent whom he loves and upon whom he depends,"[48] explains Brown.

Driving and ADHD

Learning to drive is an important milestone for most teens, but for teens with ADHD, driving can be a major challenge. Research shows that teen drivers with ADHD have higher rates of traffic tickets and accidents than teens who do not have the disorder. They are also two to four times more likely to get into an accident, a rate that makes them more likely to have a car accident than an adult driving legally drunk.

Inattention and impulsivity, hallmark symptoms of ADHD, are major factors in car accidents. Inattention is the single leading cause of car crashes among all drivers, according to Bruce Simons-Morton, a senior investigator at the National Institute for Child Health and Human Development in Bethesda, Maryland. "When a driver takes his eyes off the road for two seconds or more, he's doubled the risk of a crash,"[49] he says. For teens with ADHD who struggle with inattention, a momentary lapse in focus can lead to an accident. In addition, impulsiveness, which is linked to high levels of risk taking, can cause problems for teens

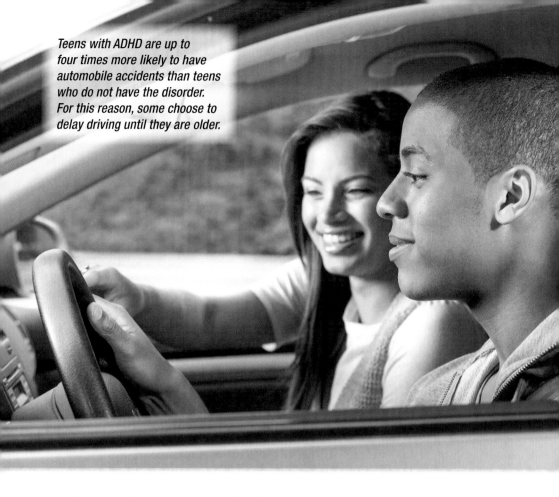

Teens with ADHD are up to four times more likely to have automobile accidents than teens who do not have the disorder. For this reason, some choose to delay driving until they are older.

in the car. They may speed, change lanes quickly, or take other thrill-seeking risks while driving. The combination of inattention and impulsivity can lead to danger for teens with ADHD, making accidents and serious injury more likely. "They're more prone to crashes because of inattention, but the reason their crashes are so much worse is because they're so often speeding,"[50] says Russell A. Barkley, who has studied driving-related issues concerning teens with ADHD. In addition, Barkley notes that many drivers with ADHD overestimate how well they can drive, which can also lead to accidents.

For Jillian Serpa, learning to drive with ADHD has been frightening. When she was sixteen, Serpa's father took her out driving. Flustered by the series of instructions that her father gave her as she backed out of the driveway, she ended up driving the family car over a creek next to her home in New Jersey. "There was a lack of communication," she says. "I stepped on the gas instead of the brake."[51] The next time she tried to practice, she panicked at a busy intersection. The incidents were so unsettling that Serpa decided to hold off on driving for four years.

Risky Behavior

For many people, ADHD can lead to poor decisions and risky behaviors. Many teens, and especially those with ADHD, act first and think about consequences later. "In general, they're more impulsive. They do things without thinking," says Mark DeAntonio, a psychiatry professor at the University of California, Los Angeles. "Another thing is that they often have complaints of being easily bored. Often, what gets their attention are things that are more risky or exciting . . . and they often don't fully consider the consequences of their acts." DeAntonio says that although almost all of his teen patients deal with impulsivity, only about one-third participate in dangerous behaviors. "Some of these behaviors are things that other teens [without ADHD] do, but they're willing to push it to the limits,"[52] he says. Teens with ADHD may engage in high-risk sports such as skateboarding, surfing, or rock climbing and may have more injuries such as broken bones. Others drive recklessly, engage in unprotected sex, smoke, or use drugs and alcohol. Some teens with ADHD steal things, get into fights, and taunt others.

> "They're more prone to crashes because of inattention, but the reason their crashes are so much worse is because they're so often speeding."[50]
>
> —Russell A. Barkley of the Medical University of South Carolina, who has studied driving-related issues for teens with ADHD

Teens with ADHD are more likely to experiment with cigarettes, alcohol, and drugs and to develop substance abuse problems than other teens, according to a 2013 study from the University of Pittsburgh. Researchers followed nearly six hundred children over an eight-year period through adolescence. They found that 35 percent of adolescents with ADHD reported using one or more substances, compared to 20 percent of teens without ADHD. The teens with ADHD were also more likely to have a substance abuse or dependence problem, with 10 percent reporting they had experienced significant problems from their substance use compared to 3 percent for the teens without ADHD. Teens with the disorder were also more likely to smoke cigarettes daily than their peers, 17 percent versus 8 percent. The researchers believe that the study's results suggest that more work needs to be done to prevent substance use and abuse in teens with ADHD. "We are working hard to understand the reasons why children with ADHD have increased risk of drug abuse," says Brooke Molina, a professor of psychiatry and psychology at the university's School of Medicine and lead author of the report. "Our hypotheses, partly supported by our research and that of others, is that impulsive decision making, poor school performance, and difficulty making healthy friendships all contribute."[53]

As a teenager growing up in Ireland, Niall Greene says that he turned to drugs and alcohol to manage his ADHD. "If I'm not getting enough stimuli, I create my own stimuli," he says. By the time he was fifteen he was drinking so much that he would black out. At age eighteen he moved to New York City, where he spent most of his money on alcohol. By his early twenties he was using cocaine regularly and experimenting with the drug Ecstasy. With his drug and alcohol use, Greene could not keep a job, and nothing was stable in his life. "This is what ADHD is like," he says. "You wake up, everything's fine. And by five o'clock your life is upside down. You have to find a new job. You've been kicked out of your flat. Once one thing goes wrong, everything goes wrong."[54]

Coexisting Conditions

It is not uncommon for youth with ADHD to also have at least one other coexisting condition. According to Children and Adults with Attention-Deficit/Hyperactivity Disorder (CHADD), an ADHD advocacy and education organization, more than two-thirds of people with ADHD have at least one other coexisting condition. In many cases, the symptoms of ADHD can mask these other disorders. When one or more coexisting disorders are present, treating ADHD and its academic, behavioral, and emotional issues can be more complicated. And if left untreated, these coexisting

School Accommodations

Students with ADHD often have trouble paying attention in class, concentrating on what a teacher is saying, and completing classwork. For many students, certain accommodations that help minimize distractions can help them manage symptoms and succeed in a regular school setting. Sitting near the teacher and away from windows and doors can help a student stay focused on what the teacher is saying. Because many students with ADHD have trouble remembering verbal instructions, teachers who allow them to record the assignments can also help keep them organized. Some schools grant students extra time for taking tests or lighten their homework assignments. Hyperactive students might be allowed to run errands for the teacher, giving them a chance to get up and move in a positive way. For some students with more severe ADHD symptoms, special education services are needed. These services can happen in a regular classroom or a special classroom according to the student's needs.

conditions can cause additional problems for people with ADHD and their families.

Although many different disorders can occur with ADHD, some are more common than others. According to CHADD, about 40 percent of people with ADHD have oppositional defiant disorder (ODD), a condition marked by defiant and disobedient behavior toward authority figures. A teen with ODD may argue, lose his or her temper frequently, and refuse to follow rules. Conduct disorder may also be present in people with ADHD, occurring in 27 percent of children and 45 to 50 percent of adolescents. Teens with conduct disorder may act aggressively, destroy property, run away, or skip school. Up to half of children and teens with ADHD also have a learning disorder. Learning disorders affect how people learn and use new information. The most common learning disorders are dyslexia, which causes problems with reading, and dyscalculia, a severe difficulty in doing math calculations.

Mood disorders and anxiety are also common coexisting conditions with ADHD. According to CHADD, approximately 38 percent of people with ADHD have a co-occurring mood disorder such as depression or bipolar disorder. These disorders can cause extreme changes in mood. People may cry easily or be irritable for no particular reason. People with bipolar disorder may go through periods of extremely elevated mood and energy that alternate with low depressive periods. Up to 30 percent of children and 53 percent of adults with ADHD also suffer from anxiety. People with anxiety worry excessively, may always be on edge and stressed out, and have trouble sleeping.

Living with ADHD

Despite having to manage the attention, hyperactivity, and impulsivity symptoms of ADHD, many people with the condition can live normal and productive lives. In fact, a number of successful people have been diagnosed and treated for ADHD, including athletes, actors, musicians, politicians, and entrepreneurs. The list includes actor Will Smith, musician John Lennon, US president John F. Kennedy, director Steven Spielberg, and basketball star Michael Jordan. The lives of these people and many others show that having ADHD does not have to be an obstacle to achieving one's goals and dreams.

CHAPTER FOUR

Can ADHD Be Treated or Cured?

ADHD is a chronic condition. Like many other chronic illnesses, ADHD cannot be cured but can be treated. Research has shown that people with ADHD who receive appropriate treatment show significant improvement in behavior at home and at school. They also have better relationships with their family and peers. Early diagnosis and treatment, however, are vital—the earlier treatment begins, the more effective it can be.

Left untreated, ADHD can negatively affect every part of a person's life. People suffering from untreated ADHD are at an increased risk of academic, social, and emotional problems from childhood into adulthood. Untreated ADHD can affect a person's job performance, marital and family relationships, and mental health. "An interesting thing happens when people are considering whether or not to treat ADHD," says psychologist Ari Tuckman. "They will often focus on the potential risks and side effects [of treatment] but ignore the potential benefits. In other words, they ignore the risks and side effects of not treating ADHD." Tuckman explains that children and teens with untreated ADHD often do not learn essential skills such as how to control their impulses, cope with emotions, and practice basic social interaction. As adults, they have trouble catching up with peers who have already learned these skills. The result can be devastating. "For kids, [not treating ADHD carries] all the risks that parents worry about," says Tuckman. "Doing badly in school, having social struggles, greater substance use, more car accidents, less likely to attend and then graduate college. For adults, untreated ADHD also affects job performance and lifetime earnings, marital satisfaction, and the likelihood of divorce."[55]

Getting a Diagnosis

The first step in managing ADHD is getting an accurate diagnosis. Many medical and psychological conditions can cause symptoms similar to ADHD; therefore, health professionals must rule out other causes of symptoms and determine if any coexisting conditions are present. They review a person's complete medical history, along with information from parents, teachers, and other family members. Many health professionals use a checklist to rate ADHD symptoms and rule out other disabilities. With this information, they can carefully assess the person's academic, social, and emotional functioning.

If the health professional diagnoses the person with ADHD, he or she will develop a treatment plan. The type of treatment suggested will depend on the person's age and severity of symptoms. For many children and teens, treatment with a combination of behavior therapy and medication is often recommended.

> "An interesting thing happens when people are considering whether or not to treat ADHD. They will often focus on the potential risks and side effects [of treatment] but ignore the potential benefits. In other words, they ignore the risks and side effects of not treating ADHD."[55]
>
> —Ari Tuckman, a psychologist who treats patients with ADHD

Behavior Therapy

Behavior therapy is a common ADHD treatment that teaches children and teens the skills they need to control their symptoms of hyperactivity, impulsiveness, and inattention. During therapy, the patient will work on strategies to stay focused and organized or reduce disruptive behavior. Overall, the goal of behavior therapy is to increase desirable behavior and reduce unwanted behavior through the use of positive and negative consequences.

Behavior therapy is enough to allow some children and teens to succeed in school and function well at home without using medication. Most experts advocate starting behavior therapy as early as possible to give a person the best chance for success.

Treatment for ADHD

Although ADHD is highly treatable, determining the best treatment option for each individual can be complicated. Parents and children have to weigh the benefits and drawbacks of medications, behavior therapy, and alternative treatments. According to the Centers for Disease Control and Prevention, medication is the most common treatment for youth between the ages of four and seventeen. Fewer than half of young people with ADHD are receiving behavior therapy, either alone or in combination with medication.

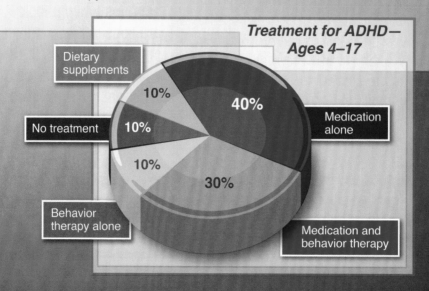

Treatment for ADHD—Ages 4–17

- Dietary supplements: 10%
- No treatment: 10%
- Behavior therapy alone: 10%
- Medication and behavior therapy: 30%
- Medication alone: 40%

Source: Centers for Disease Control and Prevention, "CDC Publishes First National Study on Use of Behavioral Therapy, Medication and Dietary Supplements for ADHD in Children," April 1, 2015. www.cdc.gov.

"These are students who enter kindergarten and first grade already behind academically and behaviorally and never quite catch up," says psychologist George J. DuPaul, chair of the department of education and human services at Lehigh University's College of Education. "Early intervention in the preschool years offers the opportunity to get a head start on trying to bridge the gap between students with attention problems and their peers."[56]

For some kids with ADHD, impulsive behavior creates problems at home and school. A type of behavior therapy called parent training can help reduce these problem behaviors, thereby enabling children to create more positive relationships with parents, teachers, and other adults in their lives. In sessions led by a clinical psychologist, parents learn how to interact with their child to encourage desired behavior and discourage disruptive behavior. Parent training teaches parents how to use praise and positive reinforcement to encourage desired behavior and how to set consistent consequences when the child does not follow instructions. The training can reduce family conflict and stress by teaching parents to react to the child's positive behavior as well as the negative. "If you think about the typical child with ADHD, they're always noticed when they're messing up," says Gregory A. Fabiano, an associate professor of counseling, school, and educational psychology at the State University of New York at Buffalo. "One of the things we try to teach adults to do is to also notice them when they're doing the right thing and then label and comment on it, so they're getting attention for good behavior."[57] This strategy has also been shown to reduce outbursts and problem behaviors at school.

Other types of behavior therapy teach kids and teens skills they need to keep up with schoolwork and manage responsibilities at home and work. This type of training is often done with learning specialists. Compared with their peers, children and teens with ADHD often have weaker executive functioning skills. This impairs their planning, organization, time-management, and decision-making skills as well as their ability to transition from activity to activity, control emotions, and learn from mistakes. Learning specialists teach specific strategies to help kids improve these skills. For example, a learning specialist might work with a young child and parents to establish routines and tools that help the child accomplish his or her work or assist the family in developing a checklist of all the steps the child must complete to get out the door for school in the morning. A rewards chart, which tracks positive behavior and allows children to earn small rewards for

> "Early intervention in the preschool years offers the opportunity to get a head start on trying to bridge the gap between students with attention problems and their peers."[56]
>
> —George J. DuPaul, chair of the Department of Education and Human Services at Lehigh University's College of Education

reaching specific goals, can motivate young kids who are easily distracted.

For teens with ADHD, time management and organization can be big challenges. Teens often underestimate how long it will take them to finish homework and projects and may forget or misplace assignments. Educational therapists might teach teens strategies to overcome these difficulties, such as using a planner to keep track of homework assignments.

Medication

For people with moderate to severe ADHD, behavior therapy might not be enough—they may need medication as well to control behavior problems and improve attention and focus. According to the CDC, about 6.1 percent of all American children take medication to treat ADHD. "I recommend medication when something causes a child to be unable to thrive in his environment,"[58] says Dr. Glen Elliott, an expert on psychoactive medications and behavioral problems in children.

Several types of medications have received approval from the Federal Drug Administration for treating ADHD. Stimulants, which have a long safety record, are the most commonly prescribed medications for this condition. People with ADHD constantly self-stimulate. They wiggle, talk all the time, and seem to be running a motor that does not turn off. Stimulant medications reduce a person's need to self-stimulate which can reduce ADHD symptoms. Stimulants work by increasing dopamine and norepinephrine in the brain, which improves concentration in people with ADHD. According to the CDC, between 70 to 80 percent of children with ADHD experience a reduction in symptoms when they take stimulant medication. Stimulants can be prescribed in immediate-release form, which allows the drug to be released into the body as soon as it is ingested. Extended-release medications, by contrast, are released into the body slowly.

While stimulant medications can be very effective at reducing ADHD symptoms, they can cause unwanted side effects. Some people taking stimulants experience sleep problems, decreased appetite, delayed growth, headaches, stomachaches, tics, and

ADHD and Diet

Some people have tried managing their diet as a way to control ADHD symptoms. In the 1970s Dr. Benjamin Feingold advised his patients to avoid certain foods. He reported that when his patients made these changes, their symptoms related to several conditions, including asthma and behavioral problems, declined. Since then, variations of Feingold's diet have been used by people hoping to improve their ADHD symptoms. Although most experts agree that diet alone is usually not enough to effectively treat ADHD, cutting back on sugary and processed foods can reduce symptoms in some people. In addition, because kids and teens on ADHD medication often have a suppressed appetite and burn a lot of calories with movement, eating a protein-rich breakfast with complex carbohydrates can fuel the body for a longer period. And adding healthy omega-3 fatty acids, found in fish or fish oil supplements, to the diet may improve ADHD symptoms.

irritability. People who experience side effects may, with the advice of their doctor, relieve them by adjusting their dosage or trying a different type of ADHD medication.

In rare cases, ADHD medications can cause more serious side effects. Some stimulants have been linked to heart and blood vessel problems, and the medications may also worsen coexisting conditions such as depression, anxiety, or psychosis. Some people, especially teens, decide to stop taking their ADHD medication to avoid the side effects. "Adherence to medication treatment is an especially important issue for adolescents with ADHD," says Eugenia Chan, a researcher at Harvard Medical School and director of the ADHD program at Boston Children's Hospital. "If they feel the medication is ineffective, causes significant side effects, or makes them feel different from their peer group, they are less likely to continue medication treatment as prescribed."[59]

Those who want to avoid the side effects of stimulants or for whom stimulant medications are not effective may be prescribed nonstimulant medications to treat ADHD. These medications also work by affecting neurotransmitters in the brain, but do not affect dopamine. One type of nonstimulant called atomoxetine, for instance, increases the amount of norepinephrine in the brain; this appears to increase attention and decrease hyperactivity and impulsiveness. Nonstimulants typically do not cause agitation or sleeplessness or suppress appetite and are often longer-lasting than stimulants. They may take longer to work than stimulants, but their effects can last up to twenty-four hours.

Although numerous ADHD groups, the American Academy of Child and Adolescent Psychiatry, and the APA recommend the use of medication for ADHD, the choice to take medication is an individual one. Many parents struggle with the decision of whether to use medication in their child's treatment. Dr. Timothy Wilens says that each child is different, and each treatment plan should consider individual circumstances. Wilens says that before prescribing medication for ADHD, he considers a child's age, the severity of symptoms, and the ways the symptoms affect the child. "If I have a child who is relatively younger, with mild symptoms, I am slower to recommend medications. I may first request environmental changes at school, or a different daily structure at school or at home," he says. "Contrast that with an 11-year-old who is struggling greatly in class, having problems paying attention, getting distracted, and becoming phobic about homework. That child is clearly on a different trajectory than what he should be and would probably benefit from medication."[60]

> "Adherence to medication treatment is an especially important issue for adolescents with ADHD. If they feel the medication is ineffective, causes significant side effects, or makes them feel different from their peer group, they are less likely to continue medication treatment as prescribed."[59]
>
> —Eugenia Chan, a researcher at Harvard Medical School and director of the ADHD program at Boston Children's Hospital

Medications affect each person differently. Whereas one person may respond well to a particular medication, another may not. Doctors may need to try different medications and dosages to find the right balance for a person. However, managing expectations are important because medication is never a cure for

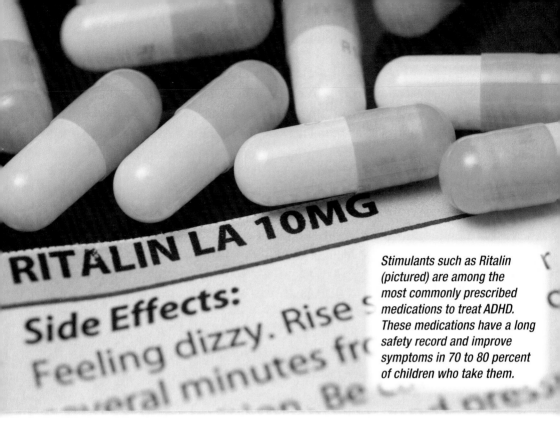

RITALIN LA 10MG

Side Effects:

Feeling dizzy. Rise s
veral minutes fro
on. Be c

Stimulants such as Ritalin (pictured) are among the most commonly prescribed medications to treat ADHD. These medications have a long safety record and improve symptoms in 70 to 80 percent of children who take them.

ADHD. It may be only one element of a combined treatment approach that also includes behavior therapy.

Alternative Treatments: Neurofeedback

Although many ADHD sufferers obtain relief from traditional behavior therapy and medication, alternative therapies are showing promise in treating symptoms—in particular the difficulty paying attention that is a hallmark of the disorder. New evidence suggests that alternative treatments that involve attention training, such as neurofeedback and mindfulness training, may help improve a person's attention and focus.

Neurofeedback uses brain exercises to increase attentiveness and reduce impulsive behavior. Neurofeedback is based on the idea of training the brain to send out signals associated with focus instead of signals associated with inattention. To begin, a patient puts on a cap lined with electrodes and performs a complex cognitive task such as reading aloud. The electrodes send signals about the brain's activity to a computer that maps the

Abuse of ADHD Medication

Although stimulant medications can greatly help students with ADHD focus and concentrate, these drugs can also be abused. According to a 2014 survey sponsored by the Partnership for Drug-Free Kids, nearly one in five college students and one in seven nonstudents aged eighteen to twenty-five abuses prescription stimulants, most commonly those prescribed for ADHD. The young adults reported that they used the drugs to stay awake, study, or perform better in school or at work.

Students who begin taking the stimulants to help them handle a heavy workload at school risk becoming addicted to the drugs. Linda Stafford, for example, was a college student in Statesboro, Georgia, when she began taking the ADHD drug Adderall without a prescription. "I wanted to go to school, work and party, and Adderall helped me to focus pretty well at first," Stafford says. Before long, though, she was addicted to the drug. She experienced depression, paranoia, and social anxiety and became cut off from family and friends. "I was totally incapable of handling life," Stafford says. "I could not manage a simple job, my class assignments or relationships. Adderall was the center of my life."

Quoted in Tara Haelle, "ADHD Stimulant Abuse Common Among Young Adults," WebMD, November 13, 2014. www.webmd.com.

areas of the brain that activated during the task and notes which areas have too much or too little brain activity. Then the patient plays a computer or video game that stimulates and rewards the areas of the brain that were identified as having too little activity. Patients receive immediate feedback as they practice focusing their attention.

In 2014 a study published in the *Journal of Pediatrics* found that children with ADHD who received neurofeedback showed more rapid and greater improvement of ADHD symptoms than children who received only behavior therapy or neither treatment. Six months after the neurofeedback sessions ended, the improvements persisted. Study researchers believe their results suggest that neurofeedback is a promising and lasting treatment for ADHD.

The experiences of Michaela's son show how effective neurofeedback can be. The boy was diagnosed with ADHD in first grade. He began taking a stimulant medication, but he still struggled with his symptoms, and although his doctors tried adjusting his medication over the years, he experienced little improvement. Then Michaela learned about neurofeedback. When her son was in sixth grade, he participated in about twenty-five neurofeedback sessions over a one-month period. "We consider neurofeedback a success," says Michaela. "At first, things got worse as his brain was reorganizing. After the second or third week, my son noted his thoughts were 'quieter than normal,' which he really liked. Overall, after a month of neurofeedback, we noticed reduced anxiety and better responses to our requests to do things he didn't like, such as homework and chores." Michaela's son was able to lower the dosage of his ADHD medication, and eighteen months after the treatment, he still shows its positive effects. "Life at home significantly improved with the treatment, while some disorganization and attentiveness are still a bit of a challenge at school,"[61] Michaela says.

One of the drawbacks to neurofeedback is the cost. Because it is considered an experimental treatment, many insurance companies do not cover it, and a course of treatment can cost $3,000 or more. "I think neurofeedback should be covered by health insurance, so this treatment would be accessible to all ADHD families and for longer treatment periods,"[62] says Michaela.

Mindful Awareness

A growing amount of research supports the idea that like neurofeedback, mindfulness exercises can help people with ADHD manage their symptoms. This approach centers around the idea of cognitive control—the ability to remain focused on an important choice, such as homework or chores, while ignoring other impulses. Typically, cognitive control increases as a child matures, with most people reaching peak levels of control in their twenties.

Many ADHD symptoms, such as poor planning, inattention, and impulsivity, are also signs of weak cognitive control. Mindfulness exercises may strengthen a person's cognitive control, helping reduce these symptoms and improving the ability to pay attention. And although taking ADHD medication can temporarily improve symptoms, some scientists believe that mindfulness training can have long-term benefits. "There are no long-term, lasting benefits from taking ADHD medications," says James M. Swanson, a psychologist at the University of California, Irvine. "But mindfulness seems to be training the same areas of the brain that have reduced activity in ADHD. That's why mindfulness might be so important," he says. "It seems to get at the causes."[63]

Mindfulness training teaches people to monitor their thoughts and feelings. Instead of following a distraction, they learn to recognize that their attention has shifted and then refocus their concentration. "Mindfulness practices range from brief and simple breath awareness practices such as counting the number of in-breaths from one to ten, beginning again whenever thoughts stray from the sensation of breathing, to guided body-scan meditations that progressively lead the focus on physical sensations throughout the body as a way of centering," explains Elizabeth Kriynovich, a teacher who leads mindfulness classes for staff and students at Delaware Valley Friends School near Philadelphia, Pennsylvania. "After mindfulness training, individuals, including adolescents with ADHD, demonstrate increased capacity for this 'regulation of attention,' which is crucial to success in classroom learning,"[64] she says.

> "Mindfulness seems to be training the same areas of the brain that have reduced activity in ADHD. That's why mindfulness might be so important. It seems to get at the causes."[63]
>
> —James M. Swanson, a psychologist at the University of California, Irvine

Research supports this observation. In a 2012 study, researchers reported that after an eight-week mindfulness training course, adolescents with ADHD noticed improved attention and fewer behavioral problems. In addition, their executive functioning improved. "Our study adds to the emerging body of evidence indicating that mindfulness training for adolescents with ADHD (and their parents) is an effective approach,"[65] concludes the study's authors.

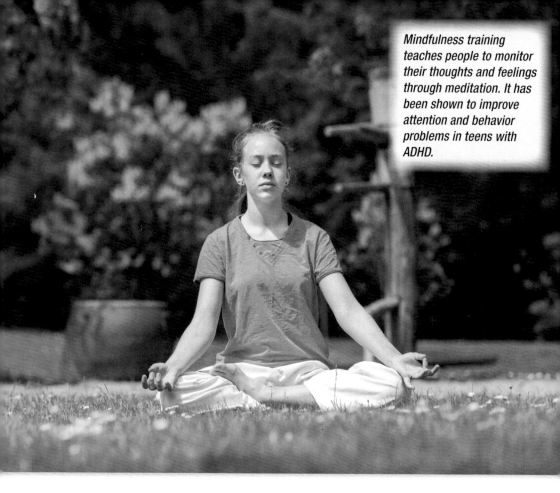

Mindfulness training teaches people to monitor their thoughts and feelings through meditation. It has been shown to improve attention and behavior problems in teens with ADHD.

Healthful Habits

In addition to traditional and alternative therapies, lifestyle habits such as eating well, exercising, and getting enough sleep can help a person reduce and manage ADHD symptoms. Many experts agree that regular exercise can help children and teens reduce ADHD symptoms. According to Matthew Pontifex, an assistant professor of kinesiology at Michigan State University, even a few minutes of physical activity each day can help people with ADHD focus better, ignore distractions, and improve their performance in school. In a 2012 study published in the *Journal of Pediatrics*, Pontifex observed the effect of exercise on forty elementary schoolchildren, half of whom had ADHD. The children spent twenty minutes walking on a treadmill or quietly reading. The group who exercised, whether they had ADHD or not, performed better on math and reading comprehension tests after the exercise. The children with ADHD who exercised were also better able to slow down and avoid mistakes on a computer game. "At the very least, exercise might be a frontline thing to consider in treatment,"[66] Pontifex says.

Getting enough sleep can also help keep ADHD symptoms under control. Even an extra half hour of sleep can reduce restlessness and improve behavior at school. On the other hand, not getting enough sleep can increase emotional outbursts, tantrums, and frustration. Studies have shown that children with ADHD can appear to be hyperactive when they are actually overly tired. "From the outside, they may look very energetic, but really it's the opposite," says Reut Gruber, an assistant professor of psychiatry and director of the Attention, Behavior, and Sleep Lab at McGill University in Canada. "It has been proposed that one reason for hyperactivity is that it helps children stay awake."[67]

Living Successfully with ADHD

Many people with ADHD manage their symptoms with a combination of therapies, medication, and healthful habits. It takes patience and commitment to live successfully with ADHD. But with persistence, people with ADHD can find the right combination of treatments to minimize their symptoms and live a full and productive life.

SOURCE NOTES

Introduction: Distracted and Unfocused

1. Quoted in John Hoffman, "What Does ADHD Really Feel Like?," Today's Parent, September 10, 2013. www.today sparent.com.
2. Quoted in Hoffman, "What Does ADHD Really Feel Like?"
3. Quoted inHoffman, "What Does ADHD Really Feel Like?"
4. Quoted in Children and Adults with Attention-Deficit/Hyperactivity Disorder, "Professional Baseball Player Shane Victorino Raises Awareness of Attention-Deficit/Hyperactivity Disorder in Young Adults and Adults Through 'Own It' Initiative," May 21, 2012. www.chadd.org.
5. Quoted in Margarita Tartakovsky, "Why ADHD Is Misunderstood," World of Psychology (blog), PsychCentral, November 27, 2014. http://psychcentral.com.
6. Quoted in Rebecca Adams, "The Common Misconception That Leaves Many Girls with ADHD Untreated," Huffington Post, December 5, 2014. www.huffingtonpost.com.

Chapter One: What Is ADHD?

7. Quoted in Wendy Donahue,"Growing Up with ADHD: Andrea's Story," Chicago Tribune, January 1, 2014. http://articles.chicagotribune.com.
8. Quoted in Jordan Lite, "A Real Mom's Story: Raising a Child with ADHD," Today, August 21, 2013. www.today.com.
9. Dana Olney-Bell, "ADHD and Me," ADDitude Magazine. www.additudemag.com.
10. Quoted in Denise Foley, "Growing Up with ADHD," Time. http://time.com.
11. Quoted in Foley, "Growing Up with ADHD."
12. Quoted in Thomas E. Brown, Smart but Stuck: Emotions in Teens and Adults with ADHD. Hoboken, NJ: John Wiley & Sons, 2014.

13. Carolyn Mallon, "Falling Through the Cracks: One ADHD Girl's Story," ADHD Homestead, April 29, 2015. http://adhdhome stead.net.

14. Quoted in Rae Jacobson, "How Girls with ADHD Are Different," Child Mind Institute. http://childmind.org.

15. Quoted in *New York Times*, "Diagnoses of ADHD on the Rise for Girls and Women," February 8, 2016. http://nytlive.ny times.com.

16. Mallon, "Falling Through the Cracks."

17. Quoted in George Washington University Milken Institute School of Public Health, "New Report Finds 43 Percent Increase in ADHD Diagnosis for US Schoolchildren: Girls Showed a Sharp Rise in ADHD Diagnosis During Eight-Year Study Period," ScienceDaily, December 8, 2015. www.sciencedaily.com.

18. Quoted in NBC News, "Diagnosis of ADHD Surges in US Kids," December 8, 2015. www.nbcnews.com.

19. Quoted in Ashley Welch, "ADHD Diagnoses Skyrocket Among US Kids," CBS News, December 8, 2015. www.cbsnews .com.

20. Dimitri Christakis, "The Diagnosis Does a Disservice to Children," *New York Times*, February 1, 2016. www.nytimes.com.

21. Donna Ford, "Don't Rush to Saddle Children with the ADHD Label," *New York Times*, February 1, 2016. www.nytimes .com.

22. Quoted in Alan Schwarz, "Doctors Train to Spot Signs of ADHD in Children," *New York Times*, February 18, 2014. www.nytimes.com.

23. Quoted in Schwarz, "Doctors Train to Spot Signs of ADHD in Children."

Chapter Two: What Causes ADHD?

24. Quoted in National Human Genome Research Institute, "Researchers Identify Gene Associated with ADHD Susceptibility," 2010. www.genome.gov.

25. Quoted in Anne Trafton, "Study Reveals a Basis for Attention Deficits," MIT News, March 23, 2016. http://news.mit.edu.

26. Quoted in Trafton, "Study Reveals a Basis for Attention Deficits."

27. Russell A. Barkley, *Taking Charge of ADHD: The Complete, Authoritative Guide for Parents*. New York: Guildford, 2013, p. 85.

28. Quoted in Kennedy Krieger Institute, "Brain Imaging Study of Preschoolers with ADHD Detects Brain Differences Linked to Symptoms," June 9, 2011. www.kennedykrieger.org.

29. Quoted in Christopher Cruz, "ADHD and Brain Structure: The Disorder Affects Teens' Memories Later in Life," Medical Daily, August 28, 2015. www.medicaldaily.com.

30. Quoted in Kristin Koch, "What Causes ADHD? 12 Myths and Facts," Health.com. www.health.com.

31. Quoted in Randy Dotinga, "Smoking While Pregnant Linked to ADHD in Children," WebMD, July 21, 2014. www.webmd.com.

32. Quoted in Shereen Lehman, "Childhood ADHD Linked to Secondhand Smoke," *Scientific American*, April 3, 2015. www.scientificamerican.com.

33. Quoted in Association for Psychological Science, "Lead Exposure Linked to ADHD in Kids with Genetic Mutation," ScienceDaily, January 7, 2016. www.sciencedaily.com.

34. Quoted in Honor Whiteman, "A Very Low Birth Weight 'May Increase Risk of Later-Life Psychiatric Problems,'" Medical News Today, February 9, 2015. www.medicalnewstoday.com.

35. Quoted in Ariana Eunjung Cha, "A New Type of ADHD? Head Injuries in Children Linked to Long-Term Attention Problems," *Washington Post*, August 3, 2015. www.washingtonpost.com.

36. Quoted in St. Michael's Hospital, "Study Finds Association Between People Who Have Had a Traumatic Brain Injury, ADHD: Findings Suggest It May Be Useful to Assess TBI History During Screening, Assessment of ADHD," ScienceDaily, August 20, 2015. www.sciencedaily.com.

37. Barkley, *Taking Charge of ADHD*, p. 99.

Chapter Three: What Is It Like to Live with ADHD?

38. Grace Friedman, "Embracing My ADHD: A Teen's Perspective," *Huffington Post*, July 28, 2014. www.huffingtonpost .com.
39. Friedman, "Embracing My ADHD."
40. Quoted in Foley, "Growing Up with ADHD."
41. Brown, *Smart but Stuck*.
42. Quoted in Maureen Connolly, "How I Got Organized in Middle School," *ADDitude Magazine*. www.additudemag.com.
43. Quoted in Connolly, "How I Got Organized in Middle School."
44. Quoted in Connolly, "How I Got Organized in Middle School."
45. Lisa Aro, "The Foolproof Way to Improve Your ADHD Child's Social Skills," Everyday Health, January 21, 2014. www.every dayhealth.com.
46. Quoted in Connolly, "How I Got Organized in Middle School."
47. Brown, *Smart but Stuck*.
48. Brown, *Smart but Stuck*.
49. Quoted in John O'Neil, "Learning to Drive with ADHD," *New York Times*, March 26, 2012. www.nytimes.com.
50. Quoted in O'Neil, "Learning to Drive with ADHD."
51. Quoted in O'Neil, "Learning to Drive with ADHD."
52. Quoted in Katherine Kam, "Teens, ADHD, and Risky Behavior," ADD Resource Center, December 1, 2013. www.addrc .org.
53. Quoted in University of Pittsburgh, Health Sciences, "Large Study Shows Substance Abuse Rates Higher in Teenagers with ADHD," ScienceDaily, February 11, 2013. www.science daily.com.
54. Quoted in Leah Sottile, "The Disturbing Relationship Between Addiction and ADHD," *Vice*, October 21, 2015. www.vice .com.

Chapter Four: Can ADHD Be Treated or Cured?

55. Quoted in Penny Williams, "Children Who Don't Get ADHD Treatment Can Have Problems into Adulthood," Healthline, May 12, 2015. www.healthline.com.

56. Quoted in Rebecca A. Clay, "Easing ADHD Without Meds," American Psychological Association, February 2013. www.apa.org.

57. Quoted in Clay, "Easing ADHD Without Meds."

58. Quoted in Bonnie Berkowitz, "Should You Give Your Kids ADHD Drugs?," *Washington Post*, June 1, 2015. www.washingtonpost.com.

59. Quoted in Lisa Rapaport, "Teens with ADHD Have Special Treatment Needs," Reuters, May 10, 2016. www.reuters.com.

60. Quoted in Berkowitz, "Should You Give Your Kids ADHD Drugs?"

61. Quoted in Penny Williams, "Can Neurofeedback Help Kids with ADHD Press the Restart Button?," *Healthline*, February 3, 2015. www.healthline.com.

62. Quoted in Williams, "Can Neurofeedback Help Kids with ADHD Press the Restart Button?"

63. Quoted in Daniel Goleman, "Exercising the Mind to Treat Attention Deficits," *Well* (blog), *New York Times*, May 12, 2014. http://well.blogs.nytimes.com.

64. Elizabeth Kriynovich, "The Benefit of Mindfulness Training for Students with Learning and Attentional Challenges," Delaware Valley Friends School, January 2015. www.dvfs.org.

65. Quoted in E. Van de Weijer et al., "The Effectiveness of Mindfulness Training on Behavioral Problems and Attentional Functioning in Adolescents with ADHD," PubMed, National Center for Biotechnology Information. www.ncbi.nlm.nih.gov.

66. Quoted in Clay, "Easing ADHD Without Meds."

67. Quoted in Clay, "Easing ADHD Without Meds."

RECOGNIZING SIGNS OF TROUBLE

ADHD affects every person differently. Whereas some people appear hyperactive, others have trouble staying focused or are overly impulsive. Symptoms of ADHD generally can be grouped into three categories: hyperactivity, inattention, and impulsivity.

Hyperactivity symptoms:
- Fidgeting and squirming
- Unable to sit still in situations where sitting is expected
- Moves constantly
- Runs and climbs inappropriately
- Talks excessively
- Acts as if driven by a motor
- Difficulty playing quietly
- Easily angered

Inattention symptoms:
- Does not pay attention to details
- Makes careless mistakes
- Easily distracted
- Appears to not listen
- Has trouble remembering and following directions
- Not organized
- Unable to plan ahead and finish projects
- Gets easily bored before a task is finished
- Often loses homework, books, or other items

Impulsivity symptoms:
- Acts before thinking
- Blurts out comments and answers in class before called on by the teacher
- Has trouble waiting for his or her turn
- Frequently interrupts
- Intrudes on other people's conversations or activities
- Difficulty controlling emotions and often has temper tantrums

The following organizations offer help for teens and others suffering from ADHD as well as detailed information about this disorder.

ADDitude Magazine

108 W. Thirty-ninth St., Suite 805
New York, NY 10018
website: www.additudemag.com

The website for *ADDitude Magazine* features articles and information about ADHD. It also has links to professional resources and discussion groups for people and families dealing with ADHD.

American Academy of Child and Adolescent Psychiatry (AACAP)

3615 Wisconsin Ave., NW
Washington, DC 20016-3007
website: www.aacap.org

The AACAP is a national professional medical association dedicated to treating and improving the quality of life for children, adolescents, and families affected by mental, behavioral, or developmental disorders. The website offers fact sheets and information on ADHD and other mental illnesses.

American Psychological Association

750 First St., NE
Washington, DC 20002-4242
website: www.apa.org

The American Psychological Association represents more than 148,000 psychologists. Its website features information about many topics, including ADHD, and links to many publications.

Association for Behavioral and Cognitive Therapies (ABCT)

305 Seventh Ave., 16th Floor
New York, NY 10001
website: www.abct.org

The ABCT represents therapists who provide behavioral therapy for people who suffer from many disorders, including ADHD. The association's website features fact sheets on several conditions, including ADHD.

Attention Deficit Disorder Association (ADDA)

website: www.add.org

ADDA provides information, resources, and networking opportunities to help teens and adults with ADHD. The website features the latest news and information about ADHD along with a directory of professional resources and support groups.

Centers for Disease Control and Prevention (CDC)

1600 Clifton Rd.
Atlanta, GA 30329-4027
website: www.cdc.gov/ncbddd/adhd

The CDC's site on ADHD contains basic information about the condition, research, data and statistics, information on conferences and training, and scientific articles.

Children and Adults with Attention-Deficit/Hyperactivity Disorder (CHADD)

4601 Presidents Dr., Suite 300
Lanham, MD 20706
website: www.chadd.org

CHADD is a national nonprofit organization that provides education, advocacy, and support for individuals with ADHD. In addition to news and information, its website offers a resources section where teens can find professionals who provide services for people living with ADHD.

LD OnLine

WETA Public Television
2775 S. Quincy St.
Arlington, VA 22206
website: www.ldonline.org

LD OnLine provides up-to-date information and advice about learning disabilities and ADHD. The site features hundreds of helpful articles, multimedia presentations, monthly columns by noted experts, first-person essays, children's writing and artwork, a comprehensive resource guide, forums, and a directory of ADHD professionals.

National Center for Learning Disabilities

32 Laight St., 2nd Floor
New York, NY 10013
website: www.ncld.org

The National Center for Learning Disabilities is an advocate for children with learning and attention issues. It is a partner in Understood.org, an online resource for parents and families dealing with learning and attention issues.

FOR FURTHER RESEARCH

Books

Russell A. Barkley, *Taking Charge of ADHD: The Complete, Authoritative Guide for Parents*. New York: Guildford, 2013.

Mark Bertin, *Mindful Parenting for ADHD: A Guide to Cultivating Calm, Reducing Stress, and Helping Children Thrive*. Oakland, CA: New Harbinger, 2015.

Thomas E. Brown, *Smart but Stuck: Emotions in Teens and Adults with ADHD*. Hoboken, NJ: John Wiley & Sons, 2014.

Sharon A. Hansen, *The Executive Functioning Workbook for Teens: Help for Unprepared, Late, and Scattered Teens.* Oakland, CA: New Harbinger, 2013.

Ruth Spodak and Kenneth Stefano, *Take Control of ADHD: The Ultimate Guide for Teens with ADHD*. Waco, TX: Prufrock, 2011.

Internet Sources

Rebecca Adams, "The Common Misconception That Leaves Many Girls with ADHD Untreated," *Huffington Post*, December 5, 2014. www.huffingtonpost.com/2014/12/05/adhd-symptoms-girls-untreated_n_6271388.html.

Thomas E. Brown, "ADHD: From Stereotype to Science," October 2013. www.drthomasebrown.com/wo-content/uploads/2016/02/ADHD_From_Stereotype_article1.pdf.

Thomas E. Brown, "Growing Up with ADHD: Clinical Care Issues," *Psychiatric Times*, January 29, 2016. www.psychiatrictimes.com/adhd/growing-adhd-clinical-care-issues.

Children and Adults with Attention-Deficit/Hyperactivity Disorder, "About ADHD." www.chadd.org/Understanding-ADHD/About-ADHD.aspx.

Children and Adults with Attention-Deficit/Hyperactivity Disorder, "Fact Sheets on ADHD." www.chadd.org/Understanding-ADHD/About-ADHD/Fact-Sheets-on-ADHD.aspx.

Denise Foley, "Growing Up with ADHD," *Time*. http://time.com./growing-up-with-adhd.

Grace Friedman, "Embracing Your ADHD," ADDYTeen.com. www.addyteen.com/adhd/.

INDEX

PICTURE CREDITS

ABOUT THE AUTHOR

Carla Mooney is the author of many books for young adults and children. She lives in Pittsburgh, Pennsylvania, with her husband and three children.